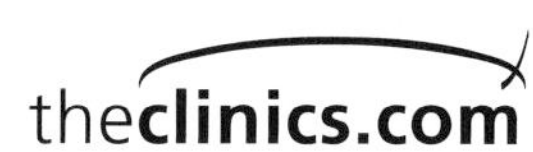


# OTOLARYNGOLOGIC CLINICS
# OF NORTH AMERICA

## Contemporary Diagnosis and Management of Head and Neck Cancer

GUEST EDITORS
Jeffrey H. Spiegel, MD, FACS
and Scharukh Jalisi, MD

February 2005 • Volume 38 • Number 1

**SAUNDERS**

An Imprint of Elsevier, Inc.
PHILADELPHIA   LONDON   TORONTO   MONTREAL   SYDNEY   TOKYO

**W.B. SAUNDERS COMPANY**
*A Division of Elsevier Inc.*

The Curtis Center • Independence Square West • Philadelphia, PA 19106–3399

http://www.theclinics.com

**THE OTOLARYNGOLOGIC CLINICS**      **Volume 38, Number 1**
**OF NORTH AMERICA**      **ISSN 0030–6665**
**February 2005**      **ISBN 1-4160-2860-9**
Editor: Molly Jay




The ideas and opinions expressed in *The Otolaryngologic Clinics of North America* do not necessarily reflect those of the Publisher. The Publisher does not assume any responsibility for any injury and/or damage to persons or property arising out of or related to any use of the material contained in this periodical. The reader is advised to check the appropriate medical literature and the product information currently provided by the manufacturer of each drug to be administered to verify the dosage, the method and duration of administration, or contraindications. It is the responsibility of the treating physician or other health care professional, relying on independent experience and knowledge of the patient, to determine drug dosages and the best treatment for the patient. Mention of any product in this issue should not be construed as endorsement by the contributors, editors, or the Publisher of the product or manufacturers' claims.


*The Otolaryngologic Clinics of North America* (ISSN 0030–6665) is published bimonthly by W.B. Saunders Company. Corporate and editorial offices: The Curtis Center, Independence Square West, Philadelphia, PA 19106–3399. Accounting and circulation offices: 6277 Sea Harbor Drive, Orlando, FL 32887–4800. Periodicals postage paid at Orlando, FL 32862, and additional mailing offices. Subscription price is $199.00 per year (US individuals), $350.00 per year (US institutions), $100.00 per year (US student/resident), $269.00 per year (Canadian individuals), $430.00 per year (Canadian institutions), $280.00 per year (international individuals), $430.00 per year (international institutions), $140.00 per year (international & Canadian student/resident). Foreign air speed delivery is included in all *Clinics'* subscription prices. All prices are subject to change without notice. POSTMASTER: Send address changes to *The Otolaryngologic Clinics of North America*, W.B. Saunders Company, Periodicals Fulfillment, Orlando, FL 32887–4800. **Customer Service: 1-800-654-2452 (US). From outside the US, call 407-345-4000.**

*The Otolaryngologic Clinics of North America* is also published in Spanish by McGraw-Hill Interamericana Editores S.A., P.O. Box 5-237, 06500 Mexico D.F., Mexico.

*The Otolaryngologic Clinics of North America* is covered in *Index Medicus, Current Contents/Clinical Medicine, Excerpta Medica, BIOSIS, Science Citation Index,* and *ISI/BIOMED.*

Printed in the United States of America.

# GUEST EDITORS

**JEFFREY H. SPIEGEL, MD, FACS,** Assistant Professor, Departments of Otolaryngology-Head and Neck Surgery and Plastic Surgery, Boston University School of Medicine; and Boston Medical Center, Boston, Massachusetts

**SCHARUKH JALISI, MD,** Clinical Instructor, Department of Otolaryngology-Head and Neck Surgery, Vanderbilt University Medical Center, Nashville, Tennessee

# CONTRIBUTORS

**DONALD J. ANNINO JR, MD, DMD,** Assistant Professor, Department of Otolaryngology, Tufts University School of Medicine, Tufts-New England Medical Center, Boston, Massachusetts

**BRIAN B. BURKEY, MD,** Vice-Chairman, Department of Otolaryngology, Vanderbilt University Medical Center, Nashville, Tennessee

**ROY R. CASIANO, MD, FACS,** Professor, Department of Otolaryngology, University of Miami School of Medicine, Miami, Florida

**FRANK CIVANTOS, MD, FACS,** Associate Professor, Department of Otolaryngology, University of Miami Hospital and Clinics/Sylvester Comprehensive Cancer Center, Miami, Florida

**SETH M. COHEN, MD, MPH,** Department of Otolaryngology, Vanderbilt University Medical Center, Nashville, Tennessee

**GEORGE L. COPPIT, MD,** Department of Otolaryngology, Walter Reed Army Medical Center, Washington, District of Columbia

**IVAN H. EL-SAYED, MD,** Clinical Instructor, Department of Otolaryngology-Head and Neck Surgery, University of California Comprehensive Cancer Center, San Francisco, California

**NANCY J. FISCHBEIN, MD,** Clinical Associate Professor of Radiology, Stanford University Medical Center, Stanford, California

**DOUGLAS K. FRANK, MD,** Attending, Department of Otolaryngology-Head & Neck Surgery, Beth Israel Medical Center, St. Luke's Roosevelt Hospital, and New York Eye & Ear Infirmary, Continuum Cancer Centers of New York; and Assistant Professor of Otolaryngology-Head & Neck Surgery, Albert Einstein College of Medicine, New York, New York

**DANIEL R. GOLD, MD,** Resident, Department of Otolaryngology, Tufts University School of Medicine, Tufts–New England Medical Center, Boston, Massachusetts

**GREGORY A. GRILLONE, MD, FACS,** Vice Chairman, Department of Otolaryngology-Head and Neck Surgery, Boston University School of Medicine, Boston, Massachusetts

**PETER HAN, MD,** Fellow, Department of Radiation Oncology, Beth Israel Medical Center and St. Luke's Roosevelt Hospital Center, Continuum Cancer Centers of New York, New York, New York

**GADY HAR-EL, MD, FACS,** Professor, Departments of Otolaryngology and Neurosurgery, State University of New York-Downstate Medical Center; and Continuum Cancer Centers, New York, New York

**LOUIS B. HARRISON, MD,** Clinical Director, Continuum Cancer Centers of New York; Chairman of Radiation Oncology, Beth Israel Medical Center and St. Luke's Roosevelt Hospital Center; and Professor of Radiation Oncology, Albert Einstein College of Medicine, New York, New York

**GRIFFITH R. HARSH, MD,** Professor of Neurosurgery and by courtesy of Otolaryngology, Stanford University Medical Center, Stanford, California

**KENNETH HU, MD,** Attending, Department of Radiation Oncology, Beth Israel Medical Center, St. Luke's Roosevelt Hospital, and New York Eye & Ear Infirmary, Continuum Cancer Centers of New York; and Assistant Professor of Radiation Oncology, Albert Einstein College of Medicine, New York, New York

**M. JALISI, FCPS, FRCS,** Former Dean, Faculty of Otolaryngology, College of Physicians and Surgeons, Pakistan; and J. J. Hospital, Karachi, Pakistan

**SCHARUKH JALISI, MD,** Clinical Instructor, Department of Otolaryngology-Head and Neck Surgery, Vanderbilt University Medical Center, Nashville, Tennessee

**SADRU KABANI, DMD, MS,** Professor and Director, Oral and Maxillofacial Pathology, Boston University Goldman School of Dental Medicine, Boston, Massachusetts

**SIDNEY P. KADISH, MD, FACR,** Professor, Department of Radiation Oncology, University of Massachusetts Medical School, Worcester, Massachusetts

**MICHAEL J. KAPLAN, MD,** Professor of Otolaryngology and Professor, by courtesy of Neurosurgery, Stanford University Medical Center, Stanford, California

**DERRICK T. LIN, MD,** Department of Otolaryngology, Massachusetts Eye and Ear Infirmary, Boston, Massachusetts

**ELIZABETH J. MAHONEY, MD,** Chief Resident, Department of Otolaryngology-Head and Neck Surgery, Boston University School of Medicine, Boston, Massachusetts

**VIKKI L. NOONAN, DMD, DMSC,** Assistant Professor, Oral and Maxillofacial Pathology, Boston University Goldman School of Dental Medicine, Boston, Massachusetts

**ROY B. SESSIONS, MD,** Chairman, Department of Otolaryngology-Head & Neck Surgery, Beth Israel Medical Center; Associate Director, Continuum Cancer Centers of New York; and Professor of Otolaryngology-Head & Neck Surgery, Albert Einstein College of Medicine, New York, New York

**MARK I. SINGER, MD, FACS,** Robert K. Werbe Distinguished Professor of Head and Neck Cancer, Department of Otolaryngology-Head and Neck Surgery, University of California Comprehensive Cancer Center, San Francisco, California

**JEFFREY H. SPIEGEL, MD, FACS,** Assistant Professor, Departments of Otolaryngology-Head and Neck Surgery and Plastic Surgery, Boston University School of Medicine; and Boston Medical Center, Boston, Massachusetts

**RANDAL S. WEBER, MD,** Professor and Chairman, Department of Otolaryngology-Head and Neck Surgery, University of Texas MD Anderson Cancer Institute, Houston, Texas

**RICHARD O. WEIN, MD,** Assistant Professor, Department of Otolaryngology and Communicative Sciences, University of Mississippi Medical Center, Jackson, Mississippi

**LAUREN B. YEAGER, BS,** Department of Otolaryngology-Head and Neck Surgery, Boston University School of Medicine, Boston, Massachusetts

# CONTENTS



> This article endeavors to explain the advantages and disadvantages of radiotherapy (RT) versus transoral laser excision (TLE) and to suggest when each modality may be employed for optimal treatment of patients with this heterogeneous group of tumors. It compares RT and TLE using the criteria of cure and local control rates, posttreatment voice quality, side effects and morbidity, cost, convenience, and salvage potential.



> This article discusses the surgical options, both open and endoscopic, developed to preserve voice, maintain swallowing, and avoid permanent tracheotomy in patients with intermediate-sized laryngeal lesions.



> Oral lesions associated with premalignant changes and malignancy present in diverse ways. This article discusses the clinical characteristics of such lesions enabling clinicians to identify classical features. Additionally, an effort is made to familiarize clinicians with the significance of red and white lesions, especially those having a high index of suspicion for oral cancer, and to alert clinicians when a biopsy is mandatory.

how best to seek a primary site and, if none is identified, how to treat these patients. This article discusses theories as to the etiology of the unknown primary tumor, diagnostic modalities highlighting the role of emerging technologies, and treatment strategies.

## Management of the Neck in Salivary Gland Carcinoma 99

Daniel R. Gold and Donald J. Annino Jr.

Major salivary gland malignancies are rare. Treatment of the primary tumor involves resection with or without postoperative radiation therapy. When there is clinical neck disease, neck dissection is performed to remove gross disease. Treatment of the N0 neck is controversial. Most centers treat the high-risk patient and perform either elective neck dissection or elective neck irradiation to eradicate residual occult disease.

## Anterior Skull Base Surgery 107

Michael J. Kaplan, Nancy J. Fischbein, and Griffith R. Harsh

This article focuses on selected key anatomic considerations in anterior skull base surgery, briefly reviews common pathologies of the paranasal sinuses, and provides an overview of surgical approaches, complications, and results.

## Endoscopic Management of Anterior Skull Base Tumors 133

Gady Har-El and Roy R. Casiano

Anterior craniofacial resection has become a standard procedure for management of lesions of the anterior skull base. During the last 2 decades, modifications of the classic anterior craniofacial resection have been reported. With the introduction of endoscopic sinus techniques and instrumentation, surgeons have begun to use endoscopic approaches for management of anterior skull base lesions. This article describes endoscopic modifications of anterior craniofacial resection.

## Sentinel Lymph Node Biopsy in Head and Neck Cancer 145

Ivan H. El-Sayed, Mark I. Singer, and Frank Civantos

Sentinel lymph node biopsy (SLNB) offers a minimally invasive technique to examine the proximal lymph node basin for micrometastases in clinically N0 necks in patients head and neck cancer. This technique has been validated in the management of breast cancer and cutaneous malignant melanoma (CMM) and is under active investigation in the management of multiple other solid tumors. SLNB is used routinely in the management of head and neck melanoma and is investigational for other cancers of the head and neck. SLNB provides prognostic information for patients with CMM and identifies those patients that may benefit from additional treatment. This article examines the history, rationale,

# FORTHCOMING ISSUES



# RECENT ISSUES



---

## The Clinics are now available online!

Access your subscription at
**www.theclinics.com**

---

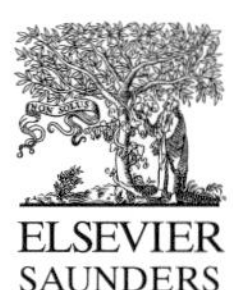

**ELSEVIER**
SAUNDERS

Otolaryngol Clin N Am
38 (2005) xiii–xiv

OTOLARYNGOLOGIC
CLINICS
OF NORTH AMERICA

Preface

# Contemporary Diagnosis and Management of Head and Neck Cancer

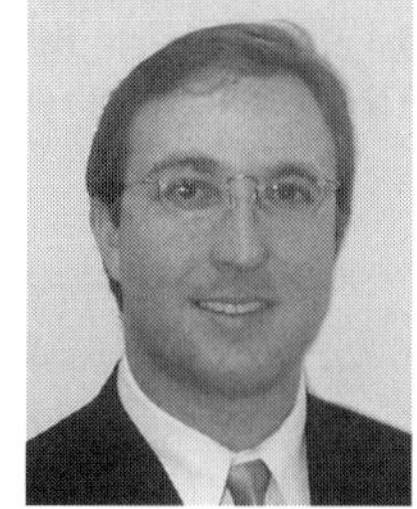

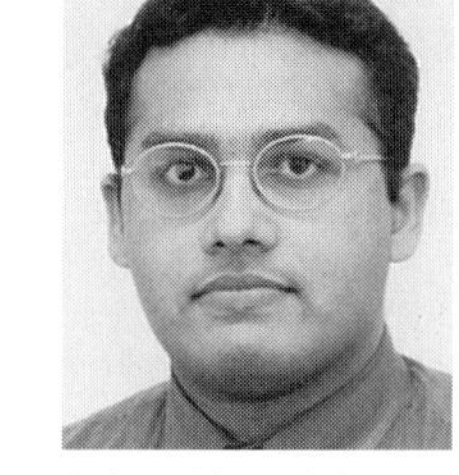

Jeffrey H. Spiegel, MD, FACS    Scharukh Jalisi, MD

*Guest Editors*

The World Cancer Report, published in 2003 by the World Health Organization, predicts an overall 50% increase in the incidence of cancer during the next 20 years. There are currently 22 million cancer patients worldwide, and another 10 million are diagnosed each year. The report goes on to suggest that cancer rates are highest and most difficult to combat in wealthier (Westernized) nations where smoking, lack of exercise, and unhealthy dietary habits are more prevalent.

Otolaryngologists are privileged to provide comprehensive care for maladies of the head and neck. Head and neck malignancy is among the most devastating disease processes we encounter, and treatment of head and neck cancer is complex. Accepted best management can vary significantly based upon seemingly subtle differences in tumor location and biology. The general otolaryngologist, who needs to be up-to-date in the management of otologic, rhinologic, laryngologic, allergy, reconstructive, and myriad other otolaryngologic topics, may find it difficult to stay current with the ever-changing literature on head and neck malignancies.

In this issue of the *Otolaryngologic Clinics of North America,* we have tried to provide a broad overview of contemporary diagnosis and management of a number of head and neck cancers. The concept for this book came during the organization of a large multidisciplinary conference held at Boston University/Boston Medical Center in June 2004 entitled, "Diagnosis & Management of Head and Neck Cancer for the Community-Based Practitioner." Several of the nationally renowned head and neck


doi:10.1016/j.otc.2004.10.013                    *oto.theclinics.com*

oncologists who have contributed to this issue have based articles on their presentations at this meeting.

We are indebted to the many talented clinicians and researchers who have devoted so much time and effort to their contributions to this text. We also wish to acknowledge the selfless support of our families and loved ones over so many years, without whom none of our efforts would see fruition.

We trust you will find the articles within to be interesting, informative, and practical. Although this issue is by no means a comprehensive text, the editors hope that the information presented here will help in refining clinical decision-making, improve the understanding of the latest surgical and nonsurgical therapies, and provide a contemporary snapshot of available treatment for our head and neck cancer patients.

Jeffrey H. Spiegel, MD, FACS
*Boston University School of Medicine*
*Department of Otolaryngology-Head and Neck Surgery*
*Boston, MA 02118, USA*

*Boston Medical Center*
*88 East Newton Street, Suite D-616*
*Boston, MA 02118, USA*

*E-mail address:* Jeffrey.Spiegel@bmc.org

Scharukh Jalisi, MD
*Vanderbilt University Medical Center*
*Department of Otolaryngology-Head and Neck Surgery*
*S-2100 Medical Center North*
*Nashville, TN 37232-2559, USA*

*E-mail address:* scharukh@hotmail.com

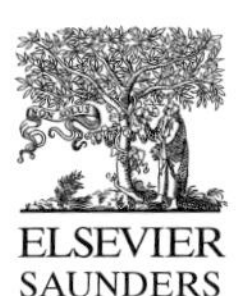

ELSEVIER
SAUNDERS

Otolaryngol Clin N Am
38 (2005) 1–9

OTOLARYNGOLOGIC
CLINICS
OF NORTH AMERICA

# Can I Treat This Small Larynx Lesion with Radiation Alone? Update on the Radiation Management of Early ($T_1$ and $T_2$) Glottic Cancer

Sidney P. Kadish, MD, FACR

*Department of Radiation Oncology, University of Massachusetts Medical School, 55 Lake Avenue North, Worcester, MA 01655, USA*

Early (T1 and T2) glottic carcinoma has been treated effectively by radiation therapy (RT) for the last half century, and, indeed, RT has been the treatment of choice. RT produces an excellent cure rate and results in near-normal to normal voice restoration. Voice quality achieved with RT is generally considered superior to that obtained with cordectomy or hemi-laryngectomy. With the introduction of transoral laser excision (TLE) during the last decade, however, this traditional judgment needs re-evaluation. TLE produces excellent cure rates and posttreatment voice quality comparable to RT in selected patients.

Because options for treatment have increased, it is important to provide clinicians some guidance. This article endeavors to explain the advantages and disadvantages of RT versus TLE and to suggest when each modality may be employed for optimal treatment of patients with this heterogeneous group of tumors. It compares RT and TLE using the criteria of cure and local control rates, posttreatment voice quality, side effects and morbidity, cost, convenience, and salvage potential.

## Staging

The American Joint Committee on Cancer (AJCC) staging for glottic carcinoma is presented in Box 1 [1]. The presence of extension to the commissure does not alter the stage designation, although some authors believe that this extension warrants a T1b designation [2]. Similarly, although the

---

*E-mail address:* KadishS@ummhc.org

0030-6665/05/$ - see front matter © 2005 Elsevier Inc. All rights reserved.
doi:10.1016/j.otc.2004.10.015

---

**Box 1. American Joint Committee on Cancer staging for glottic carcinoma [1]**

T1 Tumor limited to vocal cords (may involve anterior or
    posterior commissure) with normal motility
    T1a - Tumor extends to one vocal cord
    T1b - Tumor involves both vocal cords
T2 Tumor extends to supraglottis and/or subglottis and/or
    impaired cord mobility
T3 Tumor limited to larynx with vocal cord fixation
T4 Tumor invades through thyroid cartilage and/or other
    tissues beyond the larynx

---

AJCC system does not specify this designation, some authors designate a T2 lesion that has vocal cord mobility impairment as T2b, whereas a T2 lesion with normal vocal cord mobility is designated as T2a [3].

Thus, the AJCC system stages glottic cancer only by anatomic extent and cord mobility. It does not account for commissure extension or tumor bulk. Its measure of the depth of invasion is indirect; that is, it is an evaluation of vocal cord mobility.

The AJCC stage designation lacks the detailed description of the cord lesion that might direct the clinician to seek treatment with either TLE or RT. Therefore, the current evaluation for a laryngeal lesion should include standard direct laryngoscopy and biopsy, videostroboscopy to assess vocal fold wave motion as a gauge of the depth of invasion, and CT or MRI to assess cartilage invasion [4].

**Local control and cure**

As shown in Tables 1 and 2, RT results in a local control rate of 80% to 93% for T1 and 65% to 78% for T2 disease. These tables show single-institution series extending over many years, with each series reporting on large numbers of unselected patients. Local control rates after surgical salvage can be higher than 90%, with laryngeal preservation rates of about 90% for T1 lesions and 71% to 88% for T2 lesions.

A similar tabulation of published TLE reports (Table 3) shows smaller numbers and covers fewer years of clinical experience, reflecting the newness of the procedure and the fact that the TLE patients are highly selected. The TLE local control rate ranges from 88% to 93%, and the laryngeal preservation rate is between 93% and 100% for T1 lesions [5]; results that are comparable with the RT experience.

What factors influence these outcomes? Involvement of the anterior commissure seems to reduce the likelihood of local tumor control for both

Table 1
Local control and surgical salvage for T1 glottic carcinoma treated by radiotherapy

| Reference | Patients (N) | Initial Local Control (%) | Surgical Salvage (%) | Ultimate Local Control (%) | Larynx Preservation |
|---|---|---|---|---|---|
| Fletcher [26] | 332 | 89 | 86 | 98 | — |
| Harwood [27] | 571 | 86 | 75 | 95 | — |
| Mittal [28] | 177 | 83 | 77 | 96 | 90 |
| Amornmarm [29] | 86 | 92 | 86 | 99 | 92 |
| Mendenhall [19] | 184 | 93 | 58 | 97 | 95 |
| Wang [30] | 723 | 90 | 78 | 97 | 95 |
| Johansen [31] | 358 | 83 | 73 | 94 | 91 |
| Le [6] | 315 | 83 | 79 | 97 | 89 |
| Lee [2] | 85 | 81 | 50 | 91 | — |

*Data from* Lee DJ. Definitive radiotherapy for squamous carcinomas of the larynx. Otolaryngol Clin N Am 2002;35:1013–33.

RT [6,7] and especially for TLE [8–10], but this finding is not universally accepted [11]. For TLE, this reduction in control rate is a function of surgical exposure, and obtaining this exposure should be regarded as an advanced technique [3]. Reduced cord mobility in T2 lesions may negatively influence treatment outcome. Fraction size may also be a factor in RT outcome for irradiated patients [2]. Although local control rates are higher, with daily dose fractions above 1.8 Gy, Le [6] reported that the technical factors of fraction size, total dose, and overall treatment time are more critical for T2 disease than for T1 disease. Tumor bulk has been described as having a highly significant effect on radiation control of a T1 lesion. Reddy et al [12] reported actuarial local control rates of 91% for small tumors but of only 58% for bulky tumors. This finding supports the Shapshay [13] approach of laser excision followed by RT in larger and more invasive T1 tumors.

Table 2
Local control and surgical salvage for T2 glottic carcinoma treated by radiotherapy

| Reference | Patients (N) | Initial Local Control (%) | Surgical Salvage (%) | Ultimate Local Control (%) | Larynx Preservation |
|---|---|---|---|---|---|
| Fletcher [26] | 175 | 74 | 50 | 79 | — |
| Harwood [27] | 316 | 68 | 50 | 84 | — |
| Van den Bogaert [32] | 61 | 68 | 50 | 94 | — |
| Amornmarm [29] | 34 | 88 | 77 | 94 | 88 |
| Mendenhall [19] | 120 | 75 | 80 | 95 | 80 |
| Karim [33] | 156 | 81 | 65 | 86 | 71 |
| Wang [30] | 173 | 69 | 74 | 94 | 74 |
| Howell-Burke [34] | 114 | 68 | 74 | 92 | 72 |
| Le [6] | 83 | 67 | — | — | — |

*Data from* Lee DJ. Definitive radiotherapy for squamous carcinomas of the larynx. Otolaryngol Clin N Am 2002;35:1013–33.

Table 3
Results of TLE for T1 and T2 glottic carcinoma

| Author | Year | Patients (n) | T-stage | Survival (%) | Local Recurrence (n) | Local Recurrence (%) |
|---|---|---|---|---|---|---|
| Eckel and Thumfart [35] | 1992 | 67 | T1–T2 | 100 | 6 | 9 |
| Steiner [36] | 1993 | 130 | T1–T2 mobile | 100 | 10 | 8 |
| Rudert and Werner [37,38] | 1995 | 106 | T1–T2 | 100 | 10 | 9 |
| Spector et al [39] | 1999 | 61 | T1 | 95 | 14 | 23 |
| Peretti et al [40] | 2000 | 140 | Tis, T1, T2 | 98 | 28 | 20 |
| Moreau [41] | 2000 | 97 | T1–T2 | 97 | 0 | 0 |
| Totals | | 601 | | | 68 | 11.3 |

*From* Beitler JJ, Johnson JT. Transoral laser excision for early glottic cancer. Int J Radiat Oncol Biol Phys 2003;56(4):1063–6; with permission.

## Posttreatment voice quality

Excellent posttreatment voice quality has established RT as the treatment of choice for early glottic cancer. Does this advantage hold up in the era of laser excision? In a thorough and comprehensive review of this subject, Simpson et al [14] present data from five studies that directly compare the voice quality results after laser cordectomy and RT. In three studies no difference is appreciated, and in two other studies RT is judged better. These authors conclude that "at best, laser cordectomy is comparable to RT for the treatment of T1 squamous cell carcinomas involving the mid third of the vocal cord." Voice quality is a subjective matter, and attempts to quantify or grade outcome have not succeeded [14]. Nevertheless, McQuirt [15] notes that post-TLE voice quality declines in proportion to the amount of vocalis muscle resected. Therefore, it is not surprising that the functional outcome with RT is regarded as superior to the harsh, breathy voice of the postcordectomy or posthemilaryngectomy patient [5,14]. These procedures do not allow full glottic closure, but Zeitels [16] holds out the hope that a laryngeal reconstruction technique called "laryngoplastic phonosurgery" may restore glottic closure, and hence a proper voice, after these more extensive surgical procedures.

What are the risk factors for poor voice quality following RT for early glottis cancer? Benninger [17] identifies continued heavy smoking during RT and extensive biopsy techniques such as vocal cord stripping or excisional biopsy as factors that may degrade the postirradiation voice quality. There is also some evidence that overuse of the voice during RT may negatively affect outcome of voice [18].

## Side effects and morbidity

Radiation-induced morbidity can be divided into acute effects and chronic or late effects. The severity of radiation reaction, both acute and chronic, is a function of total dose, daily fraction size, field size, and fractionation scheme as well as T-stage.

For T1 glottic cancer, the radiation is confined to a small (6 × 6 cm) field, because there is no indication to treat the lymph nodes. At the rate of 200 cGy/fraction, this radiation results in progressive hoarseness, dysphagia, and sore throat that increase during the 6-week course but generally resolve during the month following the treatment [6]. For T2 lesions, the field is often larger, and the dose is often higher than 6600 cGy. At the University of Florida, for example, some T2 lesions are treated to 7400 cGy using a twice-daily fractionation scheme [19].

Many irradiated patients have mild or moderate laryngeal edema following treatment. Severe laryngeal edema persisting 3 months after treatment occurs in 1.5% to 4.6% of cases and could be a sign of persistent or recurrent tumor.

Conservative measures such as antibiotics, steroids, voice rest, and smoking cessation should be tried first, but biopsy must be done if edema persists [20]. Laryngeal cartilage necrosis is a rare outcome (in approximately 1% of patients) from properly fractionated moderate-dose RT [20].

TLE, as a surgical procedure, can result in postoperative morbidity. In a review of 39 TLE-treated patients, Pearson and Salassa [11] sent 12 patients home on the day of the procedure, performed 11 temporary tracheostomies, and hospitalized patients for an average of 3.3 days. Wolfensberger and Dort [9] reported persistent hoarseness in one third of the 52 TLE patients they resected. In a review of TLE using the $CO_2$ laser from Barcelona, complications were identified in 18.9% of 275 patients. These complications included local infection (0.7%), emphysema (1%), cutaneous fistula (0.3%), postoperative bleeding (8%), dyspnea (1.8%), and aspiration pneumonia/swallowing difficulty (6.1%) [21].

Ultimately, each treatment method has side effects and morbidities. These occurrences are kept to a minimum with the professional skill, judgment, and experience of the radiation oncologist and the ENT endoscopist.


## Cost

If cure and local control rates and posttreatment voice quality are equivalent for RT and TLE, and if neither treatment method causes a great deal of morbidity, how do costs compare? This information is difficult to obtain: RT involves 27 to 33 treatments, whereas TLE can be an outpatient day-surgery procedure or can involve the costs of hospitalization or re-treatment. Some authors believe that RT is more expensive than TLE [22,23], but Foote [23] reports that RT costs are similar to those of TLE but lower than those of partial vertical laryngectomy.

In the author's experience, some patients elect RT because they can continue working full-time during the entire course of treatment. The ability to continue working proves to be psychologically supportive as well as financially helpful, and it limits the societal costs of disability.

## Convenience

A routine TLE procedure conducted as day surgery is far more convenient than a 33-fraction program radiation treatment, with its attendant daily visits. This convenience, however, is reduced or eliminated once the patient is admitted, tracheostomized, or develops surgical complications, as discussed previously. The virtue of RT is that it permits the patient to remain an outpatient, able to continue employment and a nearly normal existence during a 6-week cancer-curing treatment. This consideration becomes important in the initial management decision when dealing with patients with medical comorbidities, elderly or infirm patients, and patients who have an aversion to surgery.

## Salvage potential

Can RT be used to treat patients for whom TLE has failed? No published series specifically address this question, probably because there are few failures, and many are treated with additional surgery. These patients, however, should be ideal candidates for RT. They have low-volume disease and an excellent potential for voice preservation.

Can TLE be used in the face of RT failure? Lydiatt et al [24] reported on 78 patients treated by vertical partial laryngectomy following RT failure. There was no increase in wound complications, time to decannulation, length of hospital stay, or ability to swallow. This report demonstrates that previous RT does not increase the overall complication rate and allows a voice-preserving procedure to be accomplished without special risk. Quer et al [25] reported on 24 patients in whom RT had failed and who were treated subsequently with TLE, resulting in 75% rate of voice preservation and a 76% 5-year survival rate.

As Tables 1 and 2 show, there is an 89% to 95% likelihood of larynx preservation for T1 RT failures, and a 71% to 88% likelihood for T2 RT failures. Clearly, conservative surgery including TLE can salvage RT failures and preserve the voice. Of course, total laryngectomy is the ultimate salvage procedure, but it should be reserved as a last-resort procedure.

## Summary

Both RT and TLE can offer high cure rates, satisfactory posttreatment voice quality, and acceptable short- and long-term morbidities for early glottic cancers. After careful review of the published data, the following conclusions may be reached:

---

**Box 2. Selection criteria of TLE for early glottic cancer**

1. Midcord tumors
2. No anterior commissure involvement or extension beyond midcord
3. No medical comorbidities or anesthesia risk
4. Nearly normal mucosal wave on videostroboscopy

---

1. RT continues to be the standard against which other treatment modalities are measured.
2. TLE can provide comparable cure rates and posttreatment voice quality in selected patients.
3. TLE enjoys the advantage of being a single, outpatient procedure, offering ease and brevity of effective treatment at a lower cost. Careful patient selection is the key to the initial management decision (ie, RT versus TLE). Box 2 presents the current thinking on selection criteria for TLE [10].

As the skills of the laryngeal endoscopists improve, these selection criteria may prove too confining, and larger, bulkier, and more extensive lesions may fall within the range of TLE management. Similarly, Box 3 lists selection criteria for RT.

The otolaryngologist who finds a patient with early glottic cancer is obliged to review these selection criteria carefully and offer a recommendation. The otolaryngologist should afford the patient and family an opportunity to consult with a radiation oncologist so that genuine

---

**Box 3. Selection criteria for radiotherapy for early glottic cancer**

1. Elderly or debilitated patients
2. Patients who would not tolerate or cooperate with a temporary tracheotomy
3. Patients for whom speech and voice are especially important
4. Patients who wish to avoid surgery
5. Patients with medical comorbidities or anesthesia risks
6. Local otolaryngologists lack TLE skills
7. Patients with lesions that extend beyond TLE criteria
8. Patients who are cooperative and dependable, willing and able to keep daily treatment appointments
9. Smokers who are willing to stop smoking

---

multidisciplinary input into the initial management decision is achieved. This decision may ultimately rest on the skill of the otolaryngologist and the availability and variety of endoscopic instruments and with the type of radiotherapy treatment and treatment planning equipment available to the radiation oncologist [11].

## References


[1] American Joint Committee on Cancer. Manual for staging of cancer. 5th edition. Philadelphia: Lippincott-Raven; 1997. p. 41–6.

[2] Lee DJ. Definitive radiotherapy for squamous carcinomas of the larynx. Otolaryngol Clin North Am 2002;35:1013–33.

[3] Beitler JJ, Johnson JT. Transoral laser excision for early glottic cancer. Int J Radiat Oncol Biol Phys 2003;56(4):1063–6.

[4] Flint PW. Minimally invasive techniques for management of early glottic cancer. Otolaryngol Clin North Am 2002;35:1055–66.

[5] Snow JJ, Ballenger JJ. Otorhinolaryngology/head and neck surgery. 16th edition. Hamilton (Ontario): BC Decker, Inc.; 2003. p. 273.

[6] Le QT, Fu KK, Kroll S, et al. Influence of time and fractionation on local control of $T_1$-$T_2$ glottic carcinoma. Int J Radiat Oncol Biol Phys 1997;39(1):1–2.

[7] Nozaki M, Furatu M, Murakami Y, et al. Radiation therapy for T1 glottic cancer: involvement of the anterior commissure. Anticancer Res 2000;20:1121–4.

[8] Krespi YP, Meltzer CJ. Laser surgery for vocal cord carcinoma involving the anterior commissure. Ann Otol Rhinol Laryngol 1985;94:560–4.

[9] Wolfesberger M, Dort JC. Endoscopic laser surgery for early glottic carcinoma: a clinical and experimental study. Laryngoscope 1990;98:105–9.

[10] Casiano RR, Cooper JD, Lundy DS, et al. Laser cordectomy for $T_1$ glottic carcinoma: a 10-year experience and videostroboscopic findings. Otolaryngol Head Neck Surg 1991; 104:831–7.

[11] Pearson BW, Salassa JR. Transoral laser microresection for cancer of the larynx involving the anterior commissure. Laryngoscope 2003;113(7):1104–12.

[12] Reddy SP, Mohideen N, Marks JE. Effects of tumor bulk on vocal control and survival of patients with $T_1$ glottic cancer. Radiother Oncol 1998;47(2):161–6.

[13] Shapshay SM, Hybels RL, Bohigian RK. Laser excision of early local cord carcinoma: indications, limitations and precautions. Otorhinolaryngol 1990;99(1):46–50.

[14] Simpson CB, Postma GN, Stone RE, et al. Speech outcomes after laryngeal cancer management. Otolaryngol Clin North Am 1997;30(2):189–201.

[15] McQuirt WF, Blalock D, Koufman JA, et al. Comparative voice results after laser excision or irradiation of T1 vocal cord carcinoma. Arch Otolaryngol Head Neck Surg 1994;120: 951–5.

[16] Zeitels SM, Healy GB. Laryngology and phonosurgery. N Engl J Med 2001;344:1676–9.

[17] Benninger MS, Gillen J, Thieme P, et al. Factors associated with recurrence and voice quality following radiation therapy for $T_1$ and $T_2$ glottic carcinomas. Laryngoscope 1984;94:488–94.

[18] Stoicheff ML. Voice following radiotherapy. Laryngoscope 1975;85:608–18.

[19] Mendenhall WM, Amdur RJ, Morris CG, et al. T1–T2N0 squamous cell carcinoma of the glottic larynx treatment with radiation therapy. J Clin Oncol 2001;19:4029–36.

[20] Leibel SA, Phillips TL. Textbook of radiation oncology. Philadelphia: WB Saunders; 2001. p. 508.

[21] Vilaseca-Gonzalez I, Bernal-Sprekelsen M, Blanch-Alejandro JL, et al. Complications of transoral $CO_2$ laser surgery for carcinoma of the larynx and hypopharynx. Head Neck 2003; 25(5):382–8.

[22] Brandenburg JH. Laser cordectomy versus radiotherapy: an objective cost analysis. Ann Otolrhinolaryngol 2001;110(4):312–8.

[23] Foote RL, Buskirk SJ. Has radiotherapy become too expensive to be considered a treatment option for early glottis cancer? Head Neck 1997;19(8):692–700.

[24] Lydiatt WM, Shah JP, Lydiatt KM. Conservation surgery for recurrent carcinoma of the glottic larynx. Am J Surg 1996;172(6):622–4.

[25] Quer M, Leon X, Orus C, et al. Endoscopic laser surgery in the treatment of radiation failure of early laryngeal carcinoma. Head Neck 2000;22(5):520–3.

[26] Fletcher GH. Larynx and pyriform sinus. In: Textbook of radiotherapy. 3rd edition. Philadelphia: Lea and Febinjer; 1980. p. 330–63.

[27] Harwood AR. Cancer of the larynx. The Toronto experience. J Otolaryngol Suppl 1982;11: 3–21.

[28] Mittal B, Rao DV, Marks JE, et al. Role of radiation in the management of early vocal carcinoma. Int J Radiat Oncol Biol Phys 1983;9:997–1002.

[29] Amornmarm R, Prempree T, Viravathana T, et al. A therapeutic approach to early vocal carcinoma. Acta Radiol Oncol 1985;24:321–5.

[30] Wang CC. Carcinoma of the larynx. In: Radiation therapy for head and neck neoplasms: indications, techniques and results. Chicago: Year Book Medical Publishers; 1983. p. 165–99.

[31] Johansen LV, Overgaard J, Hjelan-Hansen N, et al. Primary radiotherapy for T1 squamous cell carcinoma of the larynx: analysis of 478 patients treated from 1963 to 1985. Int J Radiat Oncol Biol Phys 1990;18:1307–13.

[32] Van den Bogaert W, Aostyn F, Van Den Schveren E. The primary treatment of advanced vocal cord cancer: laryngectomy or radiotherapy? Int J Radiat Oncol Biol Phys 1983;9: 329–34.

[33] Karim ABMF, Kralendonk JH, Yap LY, et al. Heterogeneity of stage II glottic carcinoma and its therapeutic implications. Int J Radiat Oncol Biol Phys 1987;13:313–7.

[34] Howell-Burke D, Peters LJ, Geopfert H, et al. T2 glottic carcinoma: recurrence, salvage and survival after definitive radiotherapy. Arch Otolaryngol Head Neck Surg 1990;116:830–5.

[35] Eckel HE, Thumfart WF. Laser surgery for the treatment of larynx carcinomas: indications, techniques and preliminary results. Ann Otol Rhinol Laryngol 1992;101:113–8.

[36] Steiner W. Results of curative laser microsurgery of laryngeal carcinomas. Am J Otolaryngol 1993;14:116–21.

[37] Rudert HH, Werner JA. Endoscopic resections of glottic and supraglottic carcinomas with the CO2 laser. Eur Arch Otorhinolaryngol 1995;252:146–8.

[38] Rudert H. Technique and results of transoral laser surgery for small vocal cord carcinomas. Adv Otorhinolaryngol 1995;49:222–6.

[39] Spector JG, Sessions DG, Chao KS, et al. Stage 1 (T1 N0 M0) squamous cell carcinoma of the laryngeal glottis: therapeutic results and voice preservation. Head Neck 1999;21:707–17.

[40] Peretti G, Nicolai P, Redaelli De Zinis LO, et al. Endoscopic CO2 laser excision for Tis, T1 and T2 glottic carcinomas: cure rate and prognostic factors. Otolaryngol Head Neck Surg 2000;123:124–31.

[41] Moreau PR. Treatment of laryngeal carcinomas by laser endoscopic microsurgery. Laryngoscope 2000;110:1000–6.

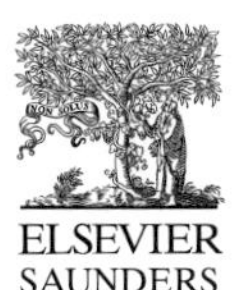

ELSEVIER
SAUNDERS

Otolaryngol Clin N Am
38 (2005) 11–20

OTOLARYNGOLOGIC
CLINICS
OF NORTH AMERICA

# Organ Preservation Surgery for Intermediate Size (T2 and T3) Laryngeal Cancer

Lauren B. Yeager, BS,
Gregory A. Grillone, MD, FACS*

*Department of Otolaryngology-Head and Neck Surgery,
Boston University School of Medicine,
88 East Newton Street, Boston, MA 02118, USA*

Before the early 1900s, cancer of the larynx was considered a fatal disease. With the advent of mass-produced cigarettes, the incidence of laryngeal cancer increased sharply, and the need for effective therapies arose. Total laryngectomy, first described by Billroth in 1873, became the mainstay of treatment for laryngeal cancers throughout the first half of the twentieth century [1]. Today, total laryngectomy remains the standard to which all other treatments are compared, but it can have significant effects on function and quality of life. Loss of the larynx is a major concern of patients, with one study showing that as many as 20% of healthy individuals would accept a decline in survival over losing the voice box [2]. Although total laryngectomy is still necessary for very large lesions, a variety of organ-preserving procedures, both open and endoscopic, has been developed to treat intermediate-sized lesions. The goal of these procedures is to preserve voice, maintain swallowing, and avoid permanent tracheotomy. This article discusses these surgical options. Although radiotherapy, with or without chemotherapy, also plays a role in the management of these lesions, these modalities are not discussed in this article.

---

* Corresponding author: Department of Otolaryngology-Head and Neck Surgery, Boston University School of Medicine, 88 East Newton Street, D-616, Boston, MA 02118.

*E-mail address:* Gregory.grillone@bmc.org (G.A. Grillone).

0030-6665/05/$ - see front matter © 2005 Elsevier Inc. All rights reserved.
doi:10.1016/j.otc.2004.10.017

*oto.theclinics.com*

## Traditional open procedures

### Vertical partial laryngectomy

In 1869 Solis-Cohen was the first to achieve a long-term cure of a glottic cancer and introduced the transcervical vertical partial laryngectomy (VPL) [3]. VPL results in a high level of control when cancer is confined to the middle third of a mobile true vocal cord. The surgery may be extended if the tumor extends anteriorly or posteriorly on the cord, spreads beyond the glottis, or results in fixed or limited mobility of the true vocal cord [4]. VPL can be performed on lesions that extend to the arytenoid, anterior commissure, or minimally onto the contralateral cord. It may also be used for tumors that extend up to 10 mm anteriorly and 5 mm posteriorly to the subglottic region [5]. VPL may be used for salvage following irradiation failure if recurrence directly correlates with the size and site of the original tumor [6]. Contraindications for VPL include involvement of the cricoarytenoid joint, involvement of more than one third of the contralateral vocal cord, and thyroid cartilage invasion [7,8].

The technique of VPL involves vertical entry into the laryngeal lumen through the thyroid cartilage. This entry can be difficult because the surgeon enters the larynx with a narrow field of exposure [4]. In standard VPL, resection extends from the anterior commissure posteriorly to include the entire membranous vocal cord and intrinsic laryngeal musculature back to the vocal process of the arytenoids and from the upper surface of the false vocal cord to about 5 mm below the edge of the true cord. A major portion of the thyroid cartilage may be resected [8]. The goal of VPL is to resect a portion of thyroid cartilage along with tumor at the glottic level [9].

Depending on tumor location, variations of VPL can be performed, and many modifications have been made in resection technique [7,9]. When tumor extends anteriorly or posteriorly on the cord, VPL with resection of the anterior commissure or paraglottic space may be performed. If cancer spreads beyond the borders of the glottis or results in fixed or limited mobility of the true vocal cord, an extended VPL should be considered. A temporary tracheotomy tube and feeding tube are required.

Reconstruction enhances postoperative voice function by replacing the soft tissue that is removed with surgery and relining the lumen of the airway with nongranulated epithelium. Various techniques have been described for the creation of the pseudocord including use of pedicled muscle flaps, bipedicled muscle flaps, and false mucosal flaps for improved voice quality [5]. Although it is important to provide enough bulk to allow the contralateral vocal cord to approximate the pseudocord, it is necessary to avoid overzealous formation of the pseudocord, which can lead to prolonged airway obstruction [10].

Most VPL patients can be decannulated within 4 to 6 weeks and are able to recover adequate swallowing function within 1 month of the procedure

[9,11]. Vocal outcome depends on reconstruction technique, but most patients are left hoarse following surgery [9].

Control rates with VPL for T2 carcinomas have been reported to be between 77% and 86% [5,12]. Glottic carcinomas that involve the anterior commissure, impair cord mobility, or extend beyond the true cord have a higher likelihood of local recurrence [5]. Laccourreye et al [13] cited recurrence rates as high as 27% to 49% when motion is impaired and as high as 11% to 50% with true vocal cord fixation.

Local control rates for T3 carcinomas remain highly variable. Failure rates greater than 30% have been reported in the literature. This high failure rate probably results from cord fixation secondary to invasion of the paraglottic space or involvement of the cricoarytenoid joint [9].

*Supraglottic laryngectomy*

As early as 1926, Felix Semon stated that 80% of supraglottic cancers could be cured by an operation less invasive than total laryngectomy [14]. Twenty years later Alonso introduced the open supraglottic laryngectomy (SGL) [15]. The procedure did not gain wide acceptance because many surgeons viewed it as oncologically unsound and because it required two stages. In 1958 Joseph Ogura [16] introduced to the United States a modified version of Alonzo's SGL that involved only a single procedure with reconstruction using skin flaps and muscle [1]. One year later Som introduced the technique of primary closure known to most otolaryngologists today [17].

SGL is a useful technique for treating intermediate-sized lesions confined to the supraglottic larynx. Patients must have good pulmonary function with a forced expiratory volume exceeding 50% [9]. SGL is contraindicated in lesions that involve the glottis, the paraglottic space, or the thyroid cartilage.

The typical supraglottic laryngectomy involves resection of the hyoid bone, epiglottis, valleculae, aryepiglottic folds, false vocal cords, and upper third of the thyroid cartilage. The procedure may be extended to include removal of part of the tongue or the pyriform sinus [18]. A temporary tracheotomy and feeding tube are required.

Reconstruction technique following SGL can vary. Typically, the tongue base is sutured to the thyroid cartilage to create a shelf of tissue overlying the glottis [9]. This overhang of tongue base tissue helps prevent aspiration during swallowing. Preservation of the hyoid bone, when oncologically feasible, allows a sturdier and more secure suspension of the larynx that results in improved swallowing function. Regardless of whether the hyoid is preserved, care must be taken during closure to ensure that the laryngeal remnant is positioned as far superior and anterior under the tongue base as possible (E. Rosen et al, grand rounds presentation, Department of

Otolaryngology, University of Texas Medical Branch, November 22, 2000) [18]. A feeding tube is generally required for 2 to 4 weeks. Voice outcome following SGL is generally good (E. Rosen et al, grand rounds presentation, Department of Otolaryngology, University of Texas Medical Branch, November 22, 2000) [19].

Aspiration can be a significant problem following supraglottic laryngectomy. Mild, temporary aspiration can occur in as many as 67% to 100% of patients (E. Rosen et al, grand rounds presentation, Department of Otolaryngology, University of Texas Medical Branch, November 22, 2000) [18]. Many patients develop low-grade chronic aspiration [19]. Postoperative rehabilitation of swallowing function is greatly facilitated by swallowing techniques, such as the "supraglottic swallow" in which patients learn to cough after each swallow. Although most patients regain adequate swallowing function following SGL, patients occasionally develop significant swallowing problems or aspiration problems requiring long-term gastrostomy feedings or total laryngectomy (E. Rosen et al, grand rounds presentation, Department of Otolaryngology, University of Texas Medical Branch, November 22, 2000).

Control rates for SGL vary in the literature depending on tumor stage and clinical nodal stage. In 1958, when Ogura [16] introduced the SGL, he reported no instance of recurrence in his initial series of patients. In the recent literature, local recurrence rates vary between 2% and 33% [1]. Bilateral neck dissection decreases the incidence of regional recurrence. Survival rates following SGL range between 64% and 76% [1,20]. The rich lymphatics of the supraglottic region predispose the patient to regional metastases and increase the risk of distant metastases that can affect survival.

## Supracricoid partial laryngectomy

Supracricoid partial laryngectomy (SCPL) was initially described in 1959 by Majer and Rieder [21] in Europe as a new open procedure designed to avoid the stigma of permanent tracheostomy associated with total laryngectomy. In spite of initial setbacks with this procedure, enthusiasm was renewed after refinements in technique by Labayle and Bismuth in 1972 [22]. Although this procedure gained wide acceptance in Europe as a useful technique to treat selected T1b, T2, and T3 supraglottic and glottic carcinomas, the procedure had not received similar recognition in the United States. Introduced to the United States in the early 1990s, the procedure has only recently begun to be accepted [9].

SCPL has been categorized into distinct procedures with unique indications and reconstruction techniques The supracricoid partial laryngectomy-cricohyoidoepiglottopexy (SCPL-CHEP) and the supracricoid partial laryngectomy-cricohyoidopexy (SCPL-CHP) are the two most common SCPL procedures performed. The former is used for glottic cancers; the latter is used for supraglottic and transglottic cancers. Other SCPL procedures include SCPL-tracheohyoidopexy and SCPL-tracheohyoidoepiglottopexy.

Indications for SCPL-CHP include T2 and T3 supraglottic carcinomas with involvement of ventricular floor, involvement of anterior commissure, impairment of vocal fold mobility, invasion of the pre-epiglottic space, or invasion of the paraglottic space. SCPL-CHEP is useful for lesions confined to the glottis, particularly those not amenable to VPL, such as bilateral glottic lesions involving a significant portion of both membranous vocal cords. Selected T4 carcinomas, transglottic carcinomas, and recurrent glottic and supraglottic cancers following radiation failure may also be indications for these procedures [9]. As with SGL, patients must have adequate pulmonary reserve. It has been shown that many patients who have undergone total laryngectomy would have been candidates for SCPL [23]. Therefore, it is important that all patients being evaluated for total laryngectomy be considered for the less radical SCPL.

Contraindications for SCPL include arytenoid cartilage fixation, posterior commissure invasion, infraglottic extent of tumor reaching the upper border of the cricoid cartilage, cricoid cartilage invasion, and extralaryngeal spread of the tumor. Invasion of the pre-epiglottic space is a contraindication for SCPL-CHEP but not for SCPL-CHP. Fixation and bilateral involvement of the vocal folds are not contraindications to this procedure as long as the arytenoid cartilage is not fixed. The exact degree of infraglottic extent that precludes surgery remains controversial [24,25]. Piquet and Chevalier [25] suggest that if there is more than 1 mm of subglottic extension, the surgery should not be performed.

SCPL is essentially an extension of SGL. SCPL-CHEP involves resection of both true vocal cords, both false vocal cords, the paraglottic spaces bilaterally, and the entire thyroid cartilage, while sparing at least one arytenoid. SCPL-CHP includes resection of the entire epiglottis and pre-epiglottic space, as well as both true vocal cords, both false vocal cords, the paraglottic spaces bilaterally, and the entire thyroid cartilage. At least one arytenoid must be spared [24].

Reconstruction following SCPL-CHP requires adequate suspension of the cricoid to the hyoid bone. With SCPL-CHEP, the cricoid must be suspended to the epiglottic remnant. During reconstruction, the pyriform sinuses and arytenoid cartilages should be positioned anteriorly to facilitate swallowing. When one arytenoid must be resected, the posterior mucosa should be preserved, if oncologically possible, to serve as a buttress for the uninvolved arytenoid.

Following SCPL, most patients can be decannulated within several weeks. Stenosis of the airway is rare but can occur. It is more common in women because of the smaller diameter of the airway at the level of the cricoid cartilage; it is also more common in patients who have been previously irradiated [9]. Stenosis in the airway may result in delayed decannulation.

The amount of rehabilitation necessary to recover adequate swallowing function depends on the extent of resection and perioperative factors, including the requirement for pre- and postoperative radiation [26]. Most patients regain adequate swallowing function after SCPL [11]. Laccoureye et al [27] reported that 98.6% of patients who had postoperative swallowing rehabilitation had normal swallowing in 6 months. Intractable aspiration is a rare but potentially devastating complication and may result in prolonged tracheotomy, prolonged feeding gastrostomy, or the need for completion laryngectomy.

Although preservation of one or both arytenoids serves as a shunt that allows voice production, the removal of the membranous vocal cord results in abnormal voice quality. Nevertheless, voice quality following SCPL is often sufficient for social interaction [18].

SCPL patients report better quality of life than patients undergoing total laryngectomy. In one study by Weinstein [23], SCPL patients scored higher on physical functioning, social functioning, physical health, and general health. They also reported greater vitality, decreased physical limitations, decreased pain, and better voice quality than total laryngectomy patients.

Local control and survival rates for SCPL are comparable with those for total laryngectomy [1,16]. Local control is high with SCPL because the wide resection of the paraglottic space and thyroid cartilage results in safe dissection margins [6,13]. Local control rates range between 66% and 100% [9,13,23,24]. Adherence to indications is critical to obtain high rates of local control. If recurrence does occur, patients may undergo salvage total laryngectomy. Local control with salvage total laryngectomy after a failed SCPL ranges from 80% to 97.3% [13,24]. Survival rates are similar to those of total laryngectomy, and most deaths result from second primary tumors, distant metastases, or intercurrent disease.

## Endoscopic laser approaches

Endoscopic laser surgery of the larynx originated in the United States in the late 1960s. In the 10 years before that, several advances in endolaryngeal surgery set the stage for its evolution, including the development of microlaryngeal instrumentation by Kleinsasser, the introduction of the operating microscope, the development of the $CO_2$ laser for surgical applications, and the development of a means of coupling the laser to the operating microscope. Strong, Jako, and Vaughan [28,29] pioneered the development and application of the $CO_2$ laser in a wide variety of laryngeal lesions including small, easily accessible cancers of the larynx. Over the next 20 years, significant advances in technique and instrumentation made in the United States and Europe extended the indications for endoscopic laser surgery to include selected intermediate-sized lesions of the glottis and the supraglottis.

## Endoscopic management of glottic tumors

Endoscopic surgery may be used to remove lesions of the glottis. Four basic procedures based on depth of excision have been described: (1) dissection just deep to the epithelial basement membrane in the superficial aspect of the superficial lamina propria (SLP); (2) dissection within the deep aspect of the SLP, for microinvasive cancer that is more extensive but not attached to the vocal ligament; (3) dissection between the deep lamina propria (vocal ligament) and the vocalis muscle, for lesions that are attached to the ligament but not through it; and (4) dissection within the thyroarytenoid (paraglottic) musculature, for lesions penetrating the vocal ligament and invading the vocalis muscle [30]. These procedures can be adjusted and fine-tuned as needed.

Involvement of the anterior commissure or posterolateral paraglottic space presents special challenges when the endoscopic approach is used. Recent surgical advances and refinements in endoscopic technique have resulted in better exposure, allowing tumor in this area to be removed endoscopically. Endoscopic vertical partial laryngectomy (EVPL) allows exposure of the anterior commissure or the posterolateral paraglottic space by removing the false vocal cord, the ipsilateral half of the epiglottis, and the aryepiglottic fold. The use of a wide-aperture laryngoscope can greatly facilitate visualization [3]. In addition, anterior counterpressure has been shown to improve exposure at the anterior commissure [31]. Impaired vocal fold mobility is not a contraindication to EVPL, but prognosis is poorer than when there is no impairment.

Various techniques for reconstruction of the glottis following endoscopic removal of tumor include medialization laryngoplasty, lipoinjection, and thyroid lamina subluxation for anterior keyhole defects [32]. Superficial resections of the glottis generally do not require reconstruction. As excision becomes more extensive, reconstruction becomes more difficult.

Voice quality after endoscopic excision of glottic tumors varies depending on the size of the defect and the reconstruction technique used, if any. Normal conversational voice can often be achieved, but patients sometimes have impairments including difficulty modulating pitch and loudness, increased effort to speak, and the need to take frequent breaths [11,33]. Most patients undergoing endoscopic excisions of glottic tumors, even large excisions using the EVPL approach, do not require tracheotomy or feeding tubes.

Control rates may vary depending on the cancer stage and excisional technique used. Various studies have reported control rates ranging from 63% to 97% [11,16,32]. There is conflicting opinion about how the control rate for endoscopic excision compares with that for open VPL [34,35]. Advantages of the endoscopic approach include avoidance of tracheotomy, early swallowing, shorter operating time, shorter hospitalization, and improved cost effectiveness [1].

*Endoscopic management of supraglottic tumors*

In the early twentieth century, Jackson [36,37] documented resection of a supraglottic tumor using a tubed laryngoscope and punch biopsy forceps. Technologic advances since that time, such as the introduction of the surgical microscope and general endotracheal anesthesia in the 1950s, greatly improved the precision of the endoscopic technique.

In 1978, Vaughan [29] reintroduced the possibility of using the endoscopic approach on supraglottic carcinomas. A wealth of evidence supports the use of laser surgery for glottic cancer, but literature on laser treatment for supraglottic carcinoma remains scarce. Analysis of existing small case studies as well as a few larger studies indicates a promising outlook for treatment of supraglottic cancer using the endoscopic laser technique (E. Rosen et al, grand rounds presentation, Department of Otolaryngology, University of Texas Medical Branch, November 22, 2000) [19,38]. In the past decade, advances in technique by Zeitels [19], Steiner [38], and others now permit complete removal of the supraglottis endoscopically.

In general, smaller lesions involving the suprahyoid epiglottis, aryepi-glottic fold, and false vocal folds are ideal for endoscopic excision. Lesions present on the infrahyoid epiglottis and the false vocal cord are tangentially oriented and, therefore, are more difficult to resect. As with glottic tumors, optimal exposure is critical in excising supraglottic tumors endoscopically. Most laryngoscopes have been designed for exposure of the glottis. To expose the supraglottis, a variety of bi-valved laryngoscopes has been developed [1,38]. These instruments increase the surgical working area and allow full visualization of the supraglottis.

In general, recovery of swallowing function following endoscopic supraglottic laryngectomy is better than with open procedures because the endoscopic technique preserves the sensory innervation and normal suspension of the larynx (E. Rosen et al, grand rounds presentation, Department of Otolaryngology, University of Texas Medical Branch, November 22, 2000) [19]. Most patients do not require tracheotomy or feeding tubes. As with open SGL, most patients undergoing endoscopic excision have good voice outcomes.

Control rates for endoscopic approaches are comparable with those for open surgery and radiation therapy. Various studies have shown local control rates of 75% to 89% for T2 lesions, 67% for T3 lesions, and 75% overall for patients with T1, T2, and T3 lesions [1,38].

**Summary**

During the past 60 years a number of new and innovative surgical techniques have been developed to treat intermediate-sized laryngeal cancers. The goal of all these procedures is to preserve function and improve quality of life while maintaining acceptable control and survival rates. These innovative therapies offer new hope for patients but have added to the complexity of medical decision-making for the practicing otolaryngologist. Ideally, a multidisciplinary approach, including otolaryngology, radiation oncology, medical oncology, and speech pathology, should be used in the management of these patients. All surgical and nonsurgical options should be discussed with patients, and management should be tailored to the individual needs and desires of the patient.

## References


[1] Myers E, Alvi A. Management of carcinoma of the supraglottic larynx: evolution, current concepts, and trends. Laryngoscope 1996;106(5):559–67.

[2] Gopal HV, Frankenthaler R, Fried MP. Advanced cancer of the larynx. Head and neck surgery-otolaryngology. 3rd edition. Philadelphia: Lippincott Williams & Wilkins; 2001. p. 1505.

[3] Zeitels S, Dailey S, Burns J. Technique of en block laser endoscopic frontolateral laryngectomy for glottic cancer. Laryngoscope 2004;114(1):175–80.

[4] Laccourreye O, Laccourreye H, Weinstein G, et al. Supracricoid laryngectomy with cricohyoidoepiglottopexy: a partial laryngeal procedure for glottic carcinoma. Ann Otol Rhinol Laryngol 1990;99:421–6.

[5] Biller H, Ogura J, Pratt L. Hemilaryngectomy for T2 glottic cancers. Arch Otolaryngol 1971; 93:238–43.

[6] Laccourreye O, Weinstein G, Naudo P, et al. Supracricoid partial laryngectomy after failed laryngeal radiation therapy. Laryngoscope 1996;106(4):495–8.

[7] Laccourreye O, Weinstein G, Brasnu D, et al. Vertical partial laryngectomy: a critical analysis of local recurrence. Ann Otol Rhinol Laryngol 1991;100:68–71.

[8] Shaw H. A view of partial laryngectomy in the treatment of laryngeal cancer. J Laryngol Otol 1987;101:143–54.

[9] Tufano R. Organ preservation surgery for laryngeal cancer. Otolaryngol Clin North Am 2002;35:1067–80.

[10] Weissler M. Management of complications resulting from laryngeal cancer treatment. Otolaryngol Clin North Am 1997;30(2):269–78.

[11] Samlan R, Webster K. Swallowing and speech therapy after definitive treatment for laryngeal cancer. Otolaryngol Clin North Am 2002;35:1115–33.

[12] Pradhan S, Pai P, Neeli S, et al. Transoral laser surgery for early glottic cancers. Arch Otolaryngol Head Neck Surg 2003;129(6):623–5.

[13] Laccourreye O, Laccourreye H, Brasnu D, et al. Cricohyoidoepiglottopexy for glottic carcinoma with fixation or impaired motion of the true vocal cord: 5-year oncologic results with 112 patients. Ann Otol Rhinol Laryngol 1997;106:364–9.

[14] DeSanto LW, Pearson BW, Olsen KD. Utility of near-total laryngectomy for supraglottic, pharyngeal, base of tongue, and other cancers. Ann Otol Rhinol Laryngol 1989;98:2–7.

[15] Alonso JM. Conservation surgery of cancer of the larynx. Transactions of the American Academy of Opthalmology and Otolaryngology 1947;51:633–42.

[16] Ogura JH. Supraglottic subtotal laryngectomy and radical neck dissection for carcinoma of the epiglottis. Laryngoscope 1958;68:983–1003.

[17] Som ML. Surgical treatment of a carcinoma of the epiglottis by lateral pharygotomy. Trans Am Acad Opthalmol Otolaryngol 1959;63:28–49.

[18] Scweinfurth J, Silver S. Patterns of swallowing after supraglottic laryngectomy. Laryngoscope 2000;110(8):1266–70.

[19] Zeitels S. Surgical management of early supraglottic cancer. Otolaryngol Clin North Am 1997;30(1):59–78.

[20] Ogura JH, Sessions DG, Spector GJ. Conservation surgery for epidermoid carcinoma of the supraglottic larynx. Laryngoscope 1975;85:1808–15.

[21] Majer EH, Rieder W. Technique de laryngectomie permettant de conserver la perméabilité respiratoire. (La cricohioidopexie). Ann Otolaryngol Chir Cervicofac 1959;76:677–81.

[22] Labayle J, Bismuth R. La laryngectomie totale avec reconstruction. Ann Otolaryngol Chir Cervicofac 1971;88:219–28.

[23] Weinstein G, El-Sawy M, Ruiz C, et al. Laryngeal preservation with supracricoid partial laryngectomy results in improved quality of life when compared with total laryngectomy. Laryngoscope 2001;11(2):191–9.

[24] Laccourreye O, Laccourreye L, Muscatello L, et al. Local failure after supracricoid partial laryngectomy: symptoms, management, and outcome. Laryngoscope 1998;108(3):339–44.

[25] Piquet J, Chevalier D. Subtotal laryngectomy with crico-hyoido-epiglotto-pexy for the treatment of extended glottic carcinomas. Am J Surg 1991;162:357–61.

[26] Rassekh C, Driscoll B, Seikaly H, et al. Preservation of the superior laryngeal nerve in supraglottic and supracricoid partial laryngectomy. Laryngoscope 1998;108(3):445–7.

[27] Laccourreye H, Laccourreye O, Weinstein G, et al. Supracricoid laryngectomy with cricohyoidopexy: a partial laryngeal procedure for selected supraglottic and transglottic carcinomas. Laryngoscope 1990;100:735–41.

[28] Strong MS. Laser excision of carcinoma of the larynx. Laryngoscope 1975;85:1286–9.

[29] Vaughan DW, Strong MS, Jako GJ. Laryngeal cancer. Transoral treatment utilizing the $CO_2$ lasers. Am J Surg 1978;136:490–3.

[30] Zeitels S. Phonomicrosurgical treatment of early glottic cancer and carcinoma in situ. Am J Surg 1996;172(6):704–9.

[31] Desloge R, Zeitels S. Endolaryngeal microsurgery at the anterior glottal commissure: controversies and observations. Ann Otol Rhinol Laryngol 2000;109:385–92.

[32] Zeitels S, Hillman R, Franco R, et al. Voice and treatment outcome from phonosurgical management of early glottic cancer. Ann Otol Rhinol Laryngol 2002;111:3–20.

[33] Davis R, Hadley K, Smith M. Endoscopic vertical partial laryngectomy. Laryngoscope 2004;114(2):236–40.

[34] Flint P. Minimally invasive techniques for management of early glottic cancer. Otolaryngol Clin North Am 2002;35:1055–66.

[35] Pearson B, Salassa J. Transoral laser microresection for cancer of the larynx involving the anterior commissure. Laryngoscope 2003;113(7):1104–12.

[36] Jackson C, Jackson CL. Endoscopic removal of cancer of the epiglottis. Cancer of the Larynx. Philadelphia: WB Saunders; 1939. p. 52.

[37] Jackson C. Malignant disease of the epiglottis. Peroral Endoscopy and Laryngeal Surgery. St. Louis: Laryngoscope Co; 1915. p. 438–9.

[38] Iro H, Waldfahrer F, Altendorf-Hofmann A, et al. Transoral laser surgery of supraglottic cancer: follow-up of 141 patients. Arch Otolaryngol Head Neck Surg 1998;124(11):1245–50.

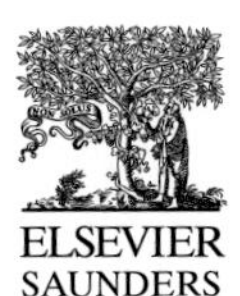

ELSEVIER
SAUNDERS

Otolaryngol Clin N Am
38 (2005) 21–35

OTOLARYNGOLOGIC
CLINICS
OF NORTH AMERICA

# Diagnosis and Management of Suspicious Lesions of the Oral Cavity

Vikki L. Noonan, DMD, DMSc*,
Sadru Kabani, DMD, MS

*Oral and Maxillofacial Pathology, Boston University Goldman School of
Dental Medicine, 100 East Newton Street, Boston, MA 02118, USA*

A change in color, texture, or consistency of the oral mucosa requires an explanation. In some instances, history and clinical presentation yield enough information for definitive diagnosis, but often biopsy with submission of lesional tissue for histologic evaluation is requisite. It is critical for a clinician to identify common oral mucosal lesions readily and to know when a specific lesion requires histologic diagnosis. The following discussion is an attempt to identify common oral mucosal changes. An effort is made to indicate key features that can be noted on clinical examination and when more invasive attempts at definitive diagnosis are indicated.

## Leukoplakia and proliferative verrucous leukoplakia

The World Health Organization defines the term "leukoplakia" (Greek for "white, flat area") as "a white patch or plaque that cannot be characterized clinically or pathologically as any other disease." The term is a clinical descriptor only; the use of the term is restricted to instances when no other diagnosis can be given based on clinical appearance alone. Upon further histologic investigation, microscopic diagnosis of clinical leukoplakic lesions can range from hyperkeratosis to dysplasia, carcinoma in situ, and invasive squamous cell carcinoma (Fig. 1).

An early study by Shafer [1] assessing the clinical characteristics of oral carcinoma in situ showed that carcinoma in situ presented clinically as a leukoplakic lesion approximately 45% of the time. Another study showed that up to 20% of leukoplakic lesions display significant epithelial alteration

---

* Corresponding author.
*E-mail address:* vnoonan@bu.edu (V.L. Noonan).

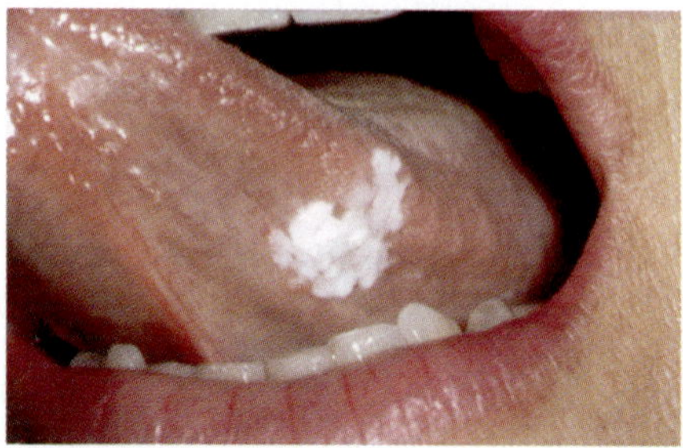

Fig. 1. Leukoplakia of lateroventral aspect of tongue. This lesion showed the entire spectrum of changes microscopically.

ranging from mild to moderate dysplasia to carcinoma in situ or invasive squamous cell carcinoma [2]. Location of a leukoplakic lesion on nonkeratinized mucosa at high-risk sites for developing oral cancer, such as the floor of the mouth, the lateral and ventral tongue, and the soft palate complex, increases the likelihood of malignant transformation [2]. Approximately two thirds of all oral cancers occur in these high-risk locations. Clinical observation indicates that one third of oral cancer cases are associated with an adjacent area of leukoplakia (Fig. 2).

One particularly persistent and importunate form of leukoplakia can be difficult to distinguish from verrucous carcinoma. Proliferative verrucous leukoplakia (PVL) is characterized as an extensive exophytic papillary proliferation that often involves multiple sites and is recalcitrant to treatment. Initial PVL lesions present in a solitary fashion characterized by thin hyperkeratosis and are well delineated from the surrounding mucosa. As the lesion evolves, it may develop a perceptually thickened quality with superficial undulations consistent with verrucous hyperplasia. The lesions become multifocal and recur following excision. Over time, the lesions progress to verrucous carcinoma or squamous cell carcinoma [3].

Unique in its predilection for women (nearly four to one over men), PVL is generally diagnosed in the seventh decade of life. Studies report that 70%

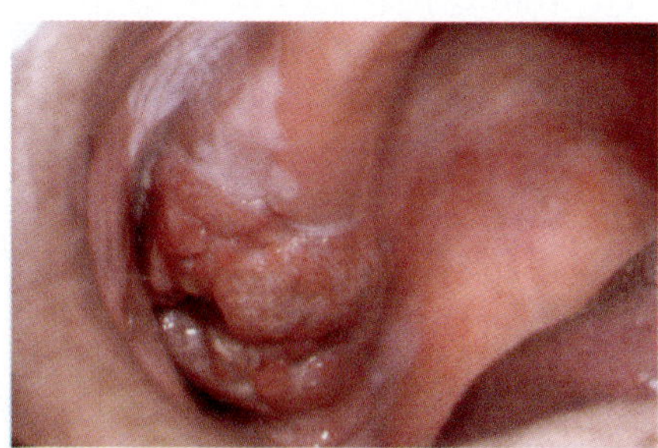

Fig. 2. Squamous cell carcinoma of the tuberosity with an adjacent area of leukoplakia.

to nearly 100% of PVL lesions progress to squamous cell carcinoma [4,5], with the gingiva and tongue being the sites showing the highest incidence of transformation [5]. Months to years may elapse from the time of initial recognition of the process to its ultimate transformation to invasive carcinoma. No apparent link between human papilloma virus and use of tobacco products has been firmly established with regard to PVL [5,6]. Given that PVL probably represents a disease that is multifactorial in nature, it is difficult to anticipate specifically who is at high risk for developing the condition.

Surgical excision is the recommended management for persistent leukoplakic lesions [7]. Recent studies have shown analysis of nuclear DNA content in leukoplakic lesions to be a useful method of prognostication in determining the capacity for a leukoplakic lesion to undergo malignant transformation [8,9]. These studies handily segregate populations of leukoplakic lesions into those that would follow a benign clinical course and those that would lead to invasive tumor based on DNA content, specifically ploidy status. Although it is too early to make meaningful conclusions, initial studies have shown that patients with leukoplakic lesions having a diploid number of chromosomes fare better than those with aneuploid leukoplakia [8,9]. Further, surgical excision of aneuploid leukoplakic lesions failed to reduce a patient's risk of eventually developing an aggressive oral cancer and dying from tumor extension [8]. This area of research may eventually change the way leukoplakic lesions are managed, so that analysis of a patient's ploidy status may be routinely used to determine if simple watchful waiting or more aggressive treatment modalities are needed to manage an oral leukoplakic lesion. Because the size of a lesion and the degree of keratinization bear virtually no correlation with histopathologic findings, clinical appearance alone can often not be relied upon as a means of definitive diagnosis. The authors' current experience indicates that white lesions, even those with benign histologic diagnoses, located at high-risk sites should be excised, and that the patient should be closely monitored at routine intervals for recurrence.

## Erythroplakia and erythroleukoplakia

Erythroplakia (Greek for "red, flat area") is a clinical term used to describe a red patch that cannot be readily classified as any other known clinical entity. Because erythematous candidiasis, nonspecific inflammatory processes, and vascular lesions may be impossible to distinguish from erythroplakia on clinical presentation alone, biopsy is required to establish a definitive diagnosis. It is not uncommon to find multiple foci of erythroplakia. Erythroplakia occurs most often on the floor of the mouth, palate, retromolar region, and tongue and generally presents in an individual in the sixth to seventh decade of life (Fig. 3) [10]. Oral erythroplakia

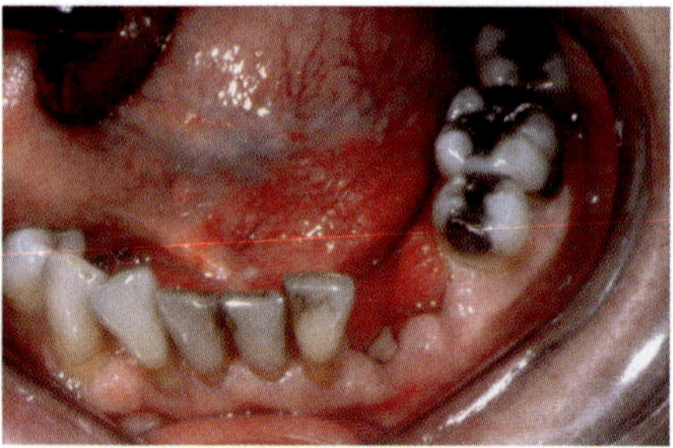

Fig. 3. Erythroplasia of the floor of the mouth. The region of two extracted teeth revealed a squamous cell carcinoma.

has a nearly 90% likelihood of representing carcinoma in situ or invasive squamous cell carcinoma at the time of diagnosis; therefore, once erythroplakia is identified, immediate action should be taken to excise the tissue in its entirety [10]. Furthermore, studies of ploidy status have indicated those erythroplakic lesions demonstrating DNA aneuploidy are at high risk of malignant transformation. Individuals with aneuploid erythroplakic lesions should be closely followed, because this finding seems to predict an increased likelihood of recurrence [11].

An early study by Shafer [1] showed approximately 16% of oral carcinoma in situ lesions were erythroplakic at the time of diagnosis and that approximately 9% were a combination of erythroplakia and leukoplakia upon clinical examination. Erythroleukoplakia represents a lesion with both red and white areas that cannot be clinically diagnosed as any other condition. Remarkable for variability in both clinical appearance and histologic findings, these mixed red and white lesions commonly show variable degrees of circumscription clinically. Additionally, histologic features of focal carcinoma in situ punctuated by areas that show normal epithelial maturation are also a hallmark finding [12]. Erythroleukoplakic lesions, therefore, require excision for thorough histologic evaluation and definitive diagnosis.

## Verrucous carcinoma

Verrucous carcinoma is a low-grade variant of squamous cell carcinoma with a characteristic papillary exophytic growth pattern (Fig. 4). A superficial neoplasm that is insidious principally because of its indolent growth course, verrucous carcinoma can be extensive and multifocal at the time of clinical presentation. Within the oral cavity, the most common sites of occurrence are the buccal mucosa and gingiva, sites typically not considered at high risk for traditional squamous cell carcinoma [13].

Although verrucous carcinoma is not confined exclusively in presentation to the upper aerodigestive tract, a significant link between oral verrucous carcinoma and tobacco products has been made [14–16]. Surgical excision is

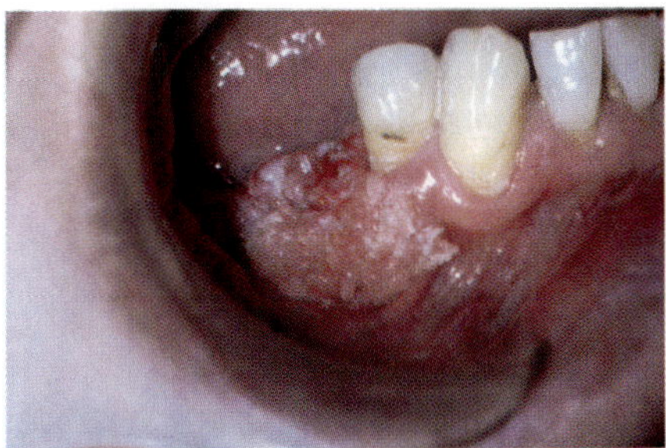

Fig. 4. Verrucous carcinoma of the alveolar ridge.

advocated as the standard of care for treatment, and many years of follow-up are required to capture additional foci because of the multicentric nature of the process and apparent increased likelihood that recurrent lesions may prove to be more poorly differentiated than their predecessor [14,16]. Further, studies have reported a nearly 20% incidence of squamous cell carcinoma arising in lesions of verrucous carcinoma. Traditional verrucous carcinoma lesions and those containing foci of invasive squamous cell carcinoma cannot be distinguished clinically [16]. This finding dictates thorough surgical excision extending deep into connective tissue to allow adequate assessment of the epithelial-connective tissue interface histologically so that multiple levels through the specimen can be subjected to histologic evaluation. Given the propensity for verrucous carcinoma to grow slowly, adequate surgical excision coupled with rigorous clinical follow-up provides the most optimistic prognosis [17].

## Squamous cell carcinoma

Oral squamous cell carcinoma, the most common intraoral malignancy, is remarkable for a variety of clinical presentations ranging from erythroplakia to leukoplakia or a combination of the two. Early lesions are generally painless. With progression, areas of ulceration and induration may be seen, and the lesion may take on increased nodularity. Fixation to underlying tissues and spread to regional lymph nodes indicates further progression to an intermediate stage of malignancy. Late-stage lesions may present with bony involvement, tooth mobility, pain, and paresthesia [18].

The use of all forms of tobacco products is associated with an increased risk of developing oral squamous cell carcinoma. When combined, tobacco and alcohol work in synergy to potentiate a markedly increased risk of developing invasive tumor [18,19]. Additionally, exposure to ultraviolet radiation (for the lip), betel quid (a mixture of slaked lime, areca nut, and tobacco wrapped in betel leaf and chewed), a social habit quite prevalent in the Indian subcontinent, and immunosuppression are well-recognized causative factors that, in a genetically susceptible individual, may yield transformation to oral squamous cell carcinoma [19].

Squamous cell carcinoma may theoretically develop in any area of the oral cavity, however, the sites most commonly involved are the posterior lateral and ventral tongue, floor of the mouth, and soft palate. Although prognosis is based largely on stage of presentation [20], it is also site dependent. For example, lesions in the posterior portion of the oral cavity have a 5-year survival rate as low as 30%, whereas carcinoma of the labial vermilion has a 5-year survival rate of approximately 70% [19]. One factor to consider when assessing these statistics is that lesions of the lip are often investigated much earlier than those presenting in the posterior region of the oral cavity. Lesions of the posterior oral cavity often present at a later stage with more challenging management issues. A final useful marker for prognostication is the presence of metastatic disease in regional lymph nodes. Positive nodal involvement reduces long-term survival by as much as 50% [20].

When an oral mucosal lesion is encountered that is suspicious in nature or is of questionable origin, an effort should be made to understand the underlying pathology. It is also important to search for synchronous or metachronous lesions, because up to 15% of patients present with "field cancerization" [21]. In their clinical review of squamous cell carcinomas of the head and neck, Sanderson and Ironside [20] list indications for immediate action in response to suspicious clinical presentation. Clinical presentations that warrant immediate action to rule out squamous cell carcinoma include nonhealing ulceration or unexplained swelling of approximately 3 week's duration and all-red or all-white lesions. In these cases, a biopsy is mandatory with definitive diagnosis by histologic examination. Additionally, it is recommended that tooth mobility unrelated to periodontal disease receive thorough investigation [20].

Most individuals afflicted with oral squamous cell carcinoma are in their fifth or sixth decade of life. Up to 75% of people with squamous cell carcinoma use tobacco products [19]. Early biopsy is recommended for any nonhealing or slowly resolving lesion, even if the patient is young and or denies exposure to tobacco products. Although extremely rare, squamous cell carcinoma has occasionally been reported in pediatric patients [22]. Additionally, recent reports have shown an increased incidence of squamous cell carcinoma in women and in patients younger than 40 years [23]. Ultimately, despite advances in treatment, prognosis depends heavily on tumor staging at the time of presentation. Thorough clinical examination and a high index of suspicion for mucosal alterations at high-risk sites provides the best chance for a positive outcome.

## Tobacco-related lesions

The use of snuff or chewing tobacco is a habit generally started before adulthood. The habit is usually modeled largely after the actions of peers

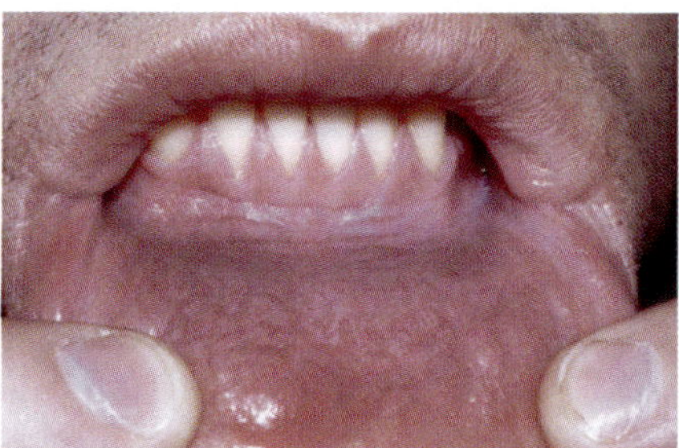

Fig. 5. Anterior mandibular mucobuccal fold with the characteristic thumb-print keratinization seen in tobacco-pouch keratosis.

and varies regionally. Although smokeless tobacco products are generally more popular among males, their use by women is increasing [24].

The long-term use of smokeless tobacco products is associated with distinct changes in the oral mucosa. One of the most worrisome oral mucosal changes produced by chronic habitual use of smokeless tobacco is leukoplakia. The leukoplakic changes associated with smokeless tobacco use are found exclusively in areas of the oral mucosa that come in direct contact with smokeless tobacco. The characteristic lesion is gray-white in color with surface fissures and indistinct borders (thumb-print appearance, Fig. 5). Other mucosal changes include gingival recession proximal to the site of tobacco placement and loss of periodontal attachment. Caries caused by chronic focal exposure to sugars in the tobacco products are also noted.

Changes in the oral mucosa following chronic smokeless tobacco use are considered premalignant changes, but the risk of developing squamous cell carcinoma from smokeless tobacco use is markedly lower than that associated with other forms of tobacco use such as cigarette smoking and betel quid chewing [25,26]. Further, an apparent risk distinction can be made based on the form of smokeless tobacco product used [26]. Still, the use of tobacco in any form should be uniformly discouraged. One hallmark feature of smokeless tobacco is the rapidity with which oral mucosal changes are induced: histologic alterations present in as few as 7 days [27]. Of clinical significance, mucosal changes usually resolve within approximately 2 weeks after cessation. Biopsy of any residual lesions is critical, because carcinomatous transformation does occur [28]. Moving the smokeless tobacco from one site to another within the oral cavity may eliminate focal areas of clinically evident leukoplakia; however doing so may extend dental complications such as periodontal disease and caries to multiple teeth at different sites.

Nicotine stomatitis, a condition related to heat generated by smoking and the consumption of hot beverages, is characterized by a fissured, "cracked mud" leukoplakic change of the hard palate punctuated by multiple erythematous nodules (Fig. 6). The erythematous nodules represent inflamed

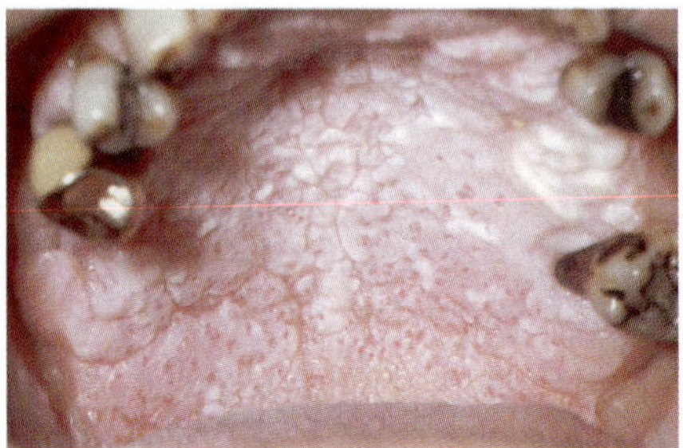

Fig. 6. Nicotine stomatitis in a long-term pipe smoker.

salivary duct orifices on the background of marked hyperkeratosis [29]. Generally not considered a premalignant condition, nicotine stomatitis probably results from the exposure of the palate to intense heat and combustion of nicotine products [30]. The oral mucosal alteration resolves quickly following cessation of the habit [29–31]. Individuals practicing the habit of reverse smoking, however, should be closely monitored because an increased risk of developing oral squamous cell carcinoma has been linked to this practice [32].

## Lichen planus, lichenoid drug reactions, and contact hypersensitivity reactions

Lichen planus is a cell-mediated mucocutaneous disorder that is remarkable for periods of exacerbation and remission. Somewhat more prevalent in women, lichen planus is present in approximately 1% to 2% of the population [33,34]. Clinically, lichen planus presents most commonly in the oral cavity in one of two forms, reticular or erosive. Multiple sites are often involved, with bilateral lesions of the buccal mucosa and lesions of the gingiva and tongue being the most common [34].

The reticular form of lichen planus is characterized by the presence of thin, interlacing linear white areas that are characteristically referred to as "Wickham's striae" after the individual who initially described this change in the late 1800s (Fig. 7). The lesions tend to wax and wane over time and are generally asymptomatic. Occasionally the lesions may have a papular or plaquelike appearance. Erosive lichen planus, on the other hand, generally elicits pain because of the formation of ulcerative regions (Fig. 8). The areas of ulceration are often circumscribed by peripheral lacey, white striae. When localized to the gingiva, the erosive form of lichen planus presents as desquamative gingivitis yielding painful areas of gingival erythema. The term "desquamative gingivitis" is clinically descriptive and may be seen in other conditions such as mucous membrane pemphigoid, pemphigus vulgaris, and hypersensitivity reactions.

Many other conditions may mimic the clinical presentation of lichen planus. Lichenoid mucositis, which is caused by a variety of stimuli, may

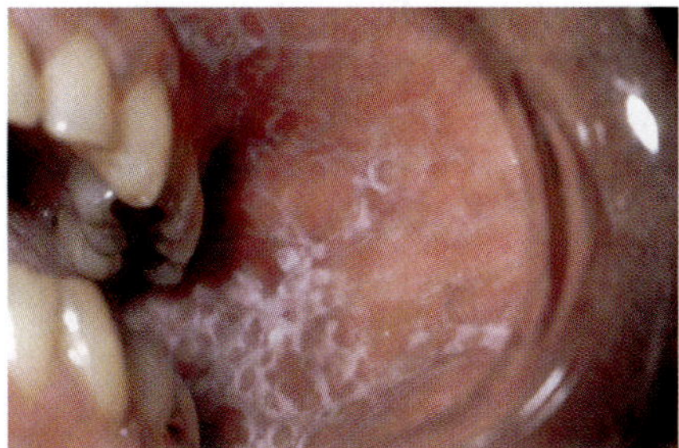

Fig. 7. Reticular/lacelike presentation of oral lichen planus. This stage is frequently asymptomatic.

superficially resemble lichen planus. For example, lichenoid reactions secondary to the use of antihypertensive medications, oral hypoglycemic agents, nonsteroidal anti-inflammatory analgesics, and antidepressant medications can produce focal reticular striae clinically indistinguishable from oral lichen planus [35,36]. Many other medications may also produce lichenoid changes. Further, focal contact hypersensitivity reactions to dental materials and flavoring agents found in chewing gum, candies, and oral hygiene products can produce so-called "lichenoid" reactions [35–37]. Cinnamon aldehyde is one such flavoring agent often implicated in the formation of lichenoid lesions. Lastly, systemic illnesses such as lupus erythematosus, chronic ulcerative stomatitis associated with autoantibodies to nuclear proteins, hepatitis C infection, and other systemic conditions such as erythema multiforme and graft-versus-host disease may present with oral lichenoid changes [35,38]. Biopsy of perilesional tissue and submission of tissue for histologic evaluation and immunofluorescence are critical. Immunofluorescence is useful in distinguishing lichen planus from chronic ulcerative stomatitis and other immune-mediated diseases. Histopathologic and immunofluorescence results combined with clinical presentation yield the most definitive diagnosis. The management of lichen planus and

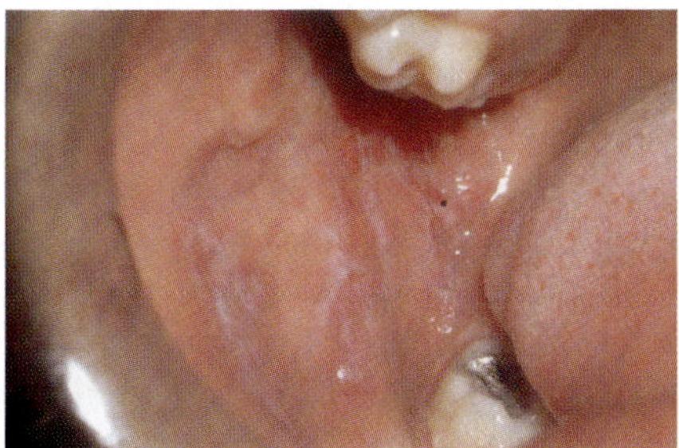

Fig. 8. Wickham's striae of buccal mucosa in lichen planus. The interspersed erythematous or erosive change may cause discomfort.

lichenoid mucositis depends largely on the severity of involvement. In the authors' experience, topical steroid gel or steroid rinses and occasional systemic steroid treatment are combined with antifungal therapy such as clotrimazole troches to prevent superimposed fungal infection and enhance healing.

The capacity for oral lichen planus to undergo malignant transformation is frequently debated in the literature. Until the relationship between oral lichen planus and malignancy is better understood, it is recommended that patients with lichenoid lesions undergo biopsy and be closely monitored at routine intervals.

## Candidiasis

Infection with *Candida albicans*, the member of the *Candida* genus most often responsible for oral candidiasis, is seen in association with immuno-suppression, antibiotic or corticosteroid treatment, smoking, chemoreductive therapy, radiation, xerostomia, and in infants who, by virtue of their immature immune system, have limited antibodies to the organism [38]. Although *Candida* can be routinely isolated from the oral cavity of healthy persons, symptomatic or clinically evident candidal infection is seen in only a percentage of these individuals [39]. Alteration of immune status, exposure to chemotherapeutic or radiation treatment, or medications may alter the oral environment in a manner that encourages overgrowth of the organism.

The classification of oral candidiasis often refers to the clinical appearance of the lesion and the acute or chronic nature of the process [40]. The simplest classification of candidiasis divides the entity into three clinical forms: pseudomembranous candidiasis, erythematous candidiasis, and hyperplastic candidiasis. Because candidiasis may present as leukoplakia, erythroplakia, or erythroleukoplakia, culture or biopsy is often necessary to confirm the diagnosis and exclude dysplasia or invasive tumor from the clinical differential. In a large percentage of patients, abnormal mucosal alterations that occur simultaneously in proximity to the candidal lesion add additional complexity to the clinical diagnostic process [41].

Pseudomembranous candidiasis (thrush) presents as multiple white plaques resembling curds of cottage cheese adhering to the oral mucosa. These plaques can be scraped away revealing an erythematous base, and the patient may complain of a burning sensation of the oral mucosa. This form of candidiasis is perhaps the most readily identified clinically and therefore is the least likely to be confused with other mucosal changes.

The erythematous form of candidiasis, on the other hand, presents a greater clinical diagnostic challenge. Typically, erythematous candidiasis presents on the dorsal tongue and palate as a red lesion with ill-defined margins that can be multifocal in nature (Fig. 9). Patients may complain of generalized oral pain or burning associated with this condition. One form of erythematous candidiasis remarkable for a distinctive presentation is

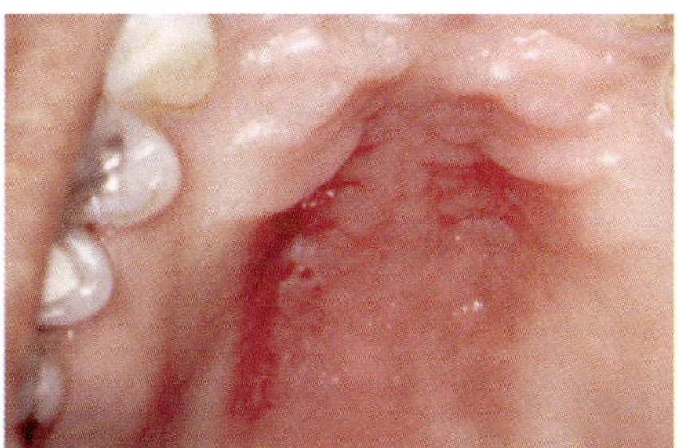

Fig. 9. The erythematous form of candidiasis.

median rhomboid glossitis. This entity is characterized by an erythematous, often nodular change secondary to filiform papillary atrophy on the posterior aspect of the mid-dorsal tongue just anterior to the circumvallate papillae. Occasionally, palatal candidiasis or so-called "kissing" lesions secondary to intimate contact with the infected dorsal tongue may be seen [42].

Finally, hyperplastic candidiasis characteristically presents on the dorsal or lateral tongue or retrocommissural region as a white plaque on clinical examination and is present with some frequency in smokers (Fig. 10). Difficult to discern from leukoplakia, hyperplastic candidiasis cannot be scraped off and is often refractory to conventional treatment with antifungal medications. Because candidal infection is often impossible to distinguish from premalignant or malignant lesions, and because its presentation is often complicated by the presence of other local or systemic disease, a biopsy of suspected candidiasis with submission for histologic evaluation together with clinical findings is recommended for definitive diagnosis [41].

## Traumatic and reactive lesions

Many lesions of the oral mucosa are caused by accidental trauma, factitial injury, or exposure to exogenous substances such as dentifrice, chemicals, or medications. One such lesion, a traumatic ulcerative granuloma

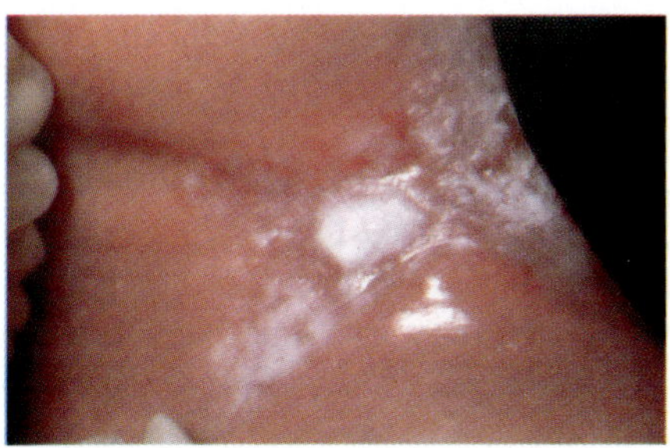

Fig. 10. The hyperplastic form of candidiasis in the retrocommissural area is indistinguishable from leukoplakia.

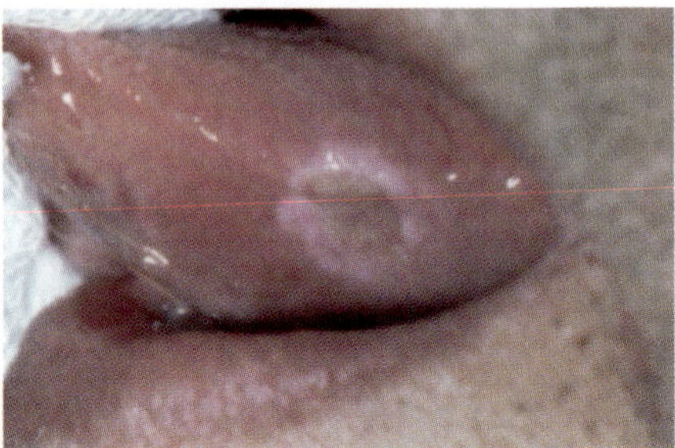

Fig. 11. A craterlike ulcer of the lateral border of the tongue with a surrounding white rim usually indicative of reactive changes.

with stromal eosinophilia (TUGSE), may be difficult to distinguish from suspected malignancy. Generally presenting on the lateral tongue or buccal mucosa following trauma (eg, bite injury), a TUGSE lesion presents as a painful "punched-out" area of ulceration that is slow to heal [43]. A white rim of hyperkeratosis and epithelial hyperplasia, a change that often indicates a reactive rather than neoplastic process, frequently surrounds the area of ulceration (Fig. 11). Because TUGSE lesions are nonhealing ulcerations often presenting at sites in the oral cavity at high risk for developing malignancy, a biopsy is frequently required to confirm the diagnosis. The lesion usually heals following the biopsy, and further treatment is not indicated.

Another oral mucosal lesion, frictional keratosis, is important to distinguish from leukoplakia. Frictional keratosis is a white lesion often found on edentulous alveolar ridge areas. This change may be present underneath a removable partial or complete denture or on an edentulous area that has not been restored and is used for mastication. Presenting as a rough, hyperkeratotic area, frictional keratosis represents a reactive epithelial response to trauma from mastication. No treatment is generally recommended for frictional keratosis unless the character of the lesion indicates otherwise, at which point the lesion may be biopsied.

Secondary to factitial injury, specifically a chronic cheek-nibbling habit, morsicatio (Latin for "bite") buccarum is another common oral mucosal change. More often seen in individuals in or beyond their fourth decade of life or in individuals undergoing some manner of psychologic stress, morsicatio typically presents as an irregular, shaggy lesion of the bilateral buccal mucosa (Fig. 12). Occasionally, lesions can also be found on the labial mucosa (morsicatio labiorum) or the lateral tongue borders (morsicatio linguarum). In many instances, the diagnosis is simplified by a characteristic clinical appearance together with a history of chronic cheek chewing. It is common, however, for an individual to be unaware of or to deny the habit. In this instance, or when a lesion presents in an atypical fashion, a biopsy may be indicated to confirm the diagnosis.

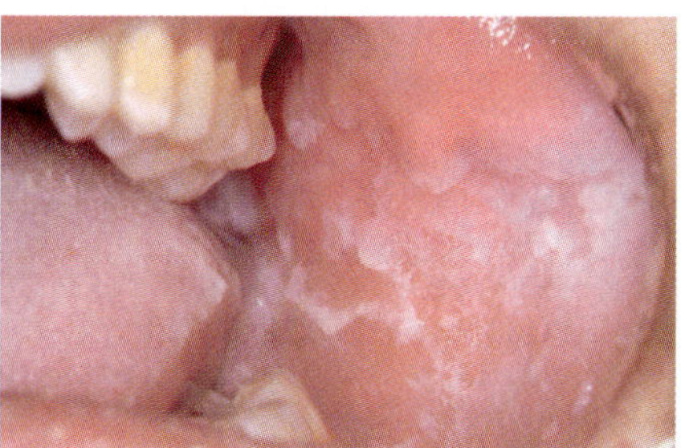

Fig. 12. Shaggy appearance caused by habitual cheek biting (morsicatio) of the buccal mucosa.

Exposure of the oral cavity to chemical substances, medications, or dentifrice can lead to specific mucosal changes. Chronic use of mouth rinses containing sanguinaria extract, a product of the bloodroot plant, can produce dysplastic leukoplakic lesions with an implied potential for malignant transformation [44]. The use of Viadent brand mouth rinse (Colgate Oral Pharmaceuticals, Canton, MA), which contains sanguinaria extract, has been shown to produce leukoplakic lesions of the maxillary vestibule, a site in which white lesions are uncommon. These lesions frequently persist and even recur following discontinuation of the product. Because biopsy may show areas of mild to moderate epithelial dysplasia, these patients should be kept under close surveillance. Given the apparent association between sanguinaria-containing dentifrice and dysplastic leukoplakia, individuals presenting with leukoplakic lesions and a history of exposure to Viadent should undergo biopsy and discontinue use of the product [44].

## Summary

The survival rate of patients with oral squamous cell carcinoma is poor despite technological advances, increased awareness of causative factors, and ease of access to the oral environment. Therefore any deviation from normal color, texture, or consistency of the oral mucosa must be definitively explained. Clinical appearance and thorough assessment frequently reveal the cause of a specific mucosal change, but one must often use biopsy and histologic evaluation to uncover the underlying pathosis. A clinician's ability to identify common oral mucosal lesions readily and, further, to know when a specific lesion requires histologic diagnosis to understand the nature of the process behind the clinical presentation is essential to improving patient survival.

## References

[1] Shafer WG. Oral carcinoma in situ. Oral Surg Oral Med Oral Pathol 1975;39:227–38.

[2] Waldron CA, Shafer WG. Leukoplakia revisited: a clinicopathologic study 3256 oral leukoplakias. Cancer 1975;36:1386–92.

[3] Hansen LS, Olson JA, Silverman S Jr. Proliferative verrucous leukoplakia: a long-term study of thirty patients. Oral Surg Oral Med Oral Pathol 1985;60:285–98.

[4] Batsakis JG, Suarez P, El-Naggar AK. Proliferative verrucous leukoplakia and its related lesions. Oral Oncol 1999;35:354.

[5] Silverman S Jr, Gorsky M. Proliferative verrucous leukoplakia; a follow up of 54 cases. Oral Surg Oral Med Oral Pathol Oral Radiol Endod 1997;84(2):154–7.

[6] Fettig A, Pogrel MA, Silverman S Jr, et al. Proliferative verrucous leukoplakia of the gingiva. Oral Surg Oral Med Oral Pathol Oral Radiol Endod 2000;90(6):723–30.

[7] Tradati N, Grigolat R, Calabrese L, et al. Oral leukoplakias: to treat or not? Oral Oncol 1997;33(5):317–21.

[8] Sudbo J, Lippman SM, Lee JJ, et al. The influence of resection and aneuploidy on mortality in oral leukoplakia. N Engl J Med 2004;350(14):1405–13.

[9] Sudbo J, Kildal W, Risberg B, et al. DNA content as a prognostic marker in patients with oral leukoplakia. N Engl J Med 2001;344(17):1270–8.

[10] Shafer WG, Waldron CA. Erythroplakia of the oral cavity. Cancer 1975;36:1021–8.

[11] Sudbo J, Kildal W, Johannessen AC, et al. Gross genomic aberrations in precancers: clinical implications of a long-term follow-up study in oral erythroplakias. J Clin Oncol 2002;20(2): 456–62.

[12] Amagasa T, Yokoo E, Sato K, et al. A study of the clinical characteristics and treatment of oral carcinoma in situ. Oral Surg Oral Med Oral Pathol 1985;60:50–5.

[13] Koch BB, Trask DK, Hoffman HT, et al. National survey of head and neck verrucous carcinoma: patterns of presentation, care and outcome. Cancer 2001;92(1):110–20.

[14] Spiro RH. Verrucous carcinoma then and now. Am J Surg 1998;176(5):393–7.

[15] Ferlito A, Recher G. Ackerman's tumor (verrucous carcinoma) of the larynx: a clinicopathologic study of 77 cases. Cancer 1980;46:1617–30.

[16] Medina JE, Dichtel W, Luna MA. Verrucous-squamous carcinomas of the oral cavity: a clinicopathologic study of 104 cases. Arch Otolaryngol 1984;110:437–40.

[17] McCoy JM, Waldron CA. Verrucous carcinoma of the oral cavity: a review of forty-nine cases. Oral Surg Oral Med Oral Pathol 1981;52(6):623–9.

[18] Zakrzewska JM. Fortnightly review: oral cancer. BMJ 1999;318(7190):1051–4.

[19] Scully C, Porter S. Oral cancer. BMJ 2000;321(7253):97–100.

[20] Sanderson RJ, Ironsinde JA. Squamous cell carcinomas of the head and neck. BMJ 2002; 325(7368):822–7.

[21] Panosetti E, Luboinski B, Marmelle G, et al. Multiple synchronous and metachronous cancers of the upper autodigestive tract: a nine-year study. Laryngoscope 1989;99:1267–73.

[22] Bill T, Reddy V, Ries KL, et al. Adolescent gingival squamous cell carcinoma: report of a case and review of the literature. Oral Surg Oral Med Oral Pathol Oral Radiol Endod 2001; 91(6):682–5.

[23] Martin-Granizo R, Rodriguez-Campo F, Naval L, et al. Squamous cell carcinoma of the oral cavity in patients younger than 40 years. Otolaryngol Head Neck Surg 1997;117(3Pt 1): 268–75.

[24] Winn DM, Blot WJ, Shy CM, et al. Snuff dipping and oral cancer among women in the southern United States. N Engl J Med 1981;304:745–9.

[25] Bouquot JE, Meckstroth RL. Oral cancer in a tobacco-chewing US population—no apparent increased incidence or mortality. Oral Surg Oral Med Oral Pathol 1998;86(6): 697–706.

[26] Rodu B, Cole P. Smokeless tobacco use and cancer of the upper respiratory tract. Oral Surg Oral Med Pral Pathol Oral Radiol Endod 2002;93(5):511–5.

[27] Payne JB, Johnson GK, Reinhardt RA, et al. Histological alterations following short-term smokeless tobacco exposure in humans. J Periodont Res 1998;35(5):274–9.

[28] Kaugars GE, Mehailescu WL, Gunsolley JC. Smokeless tobacco use and oral epithelial dysplasia. Cancer 1989;64:1527–30.

[29] Thoma KH. Stomatitis nicotina and its effect on the palate. Am J Orthod 1941;27:38–47.

[30] Rossie KM, Guggenheimer J. Thermally induced 'nicotine' stomatitis. Oral Surg Oral Med Oral Pathol 1990;70:597–9.

[31] Sutherland KG. The pathology and treatment of diseases of the palate. Aust Dent J 1968;13: 111–24.

[32] Quigley LF Jr, Cobb CM, Hunt EE Sr, et al. Reverse smoking and its oral consequences in Caribbean and South American peoples. J Am Dent Assoc 1964;69:427–42.

[33] Silverman S Jr, Gorsky M, Lozada-Nur F. A prospective follow-up study of 570 patients with oral lichen planus: persistence, remission, and malignant association. Oral Surg Oral Med Oral Pathol 1985;60:30–4.

[34] Scully C, el-Kom M. Lichen planus: review and update on pathogenesis. J Oral Pathol 1985; 14:431–58.

[35] Myers SL, Rhodus NL, Parsons HM, et al. A retrospective survey of oral lichenoid lesions: revisiting the diagnostic process for oral lichen planus. Oral Surg Oral Med Oral Pathol Oral Radiol Endod 2002;93:676–81.

[36] Epstein JB, Wan LS, Gorsky M, et al. Oral lichen planus: progress in understanding its malignant potential and the implications for clinical management. Oral Surg Oral Med Oral Pathol Oral Radiol Endod 2003;96:32–7.

[37] Thormhill MH, Pemberton MN, Simmons RK, et al. Amalgam-contact hypersensitivity lesions and oral lichen planus. Oral Surg Oral Med Oral Pathol Oral Radiol Endod 2003; 95:291–9.

[38] Scully C, Porter S. Swellings and red, white and pigmented lesions. BMJ 2000;321(7255): 225–8.

[39] Arendorf TM, Walker DM. Oral candidal populations in health and disease. Br Dent J 1979; 147:267–72.

[40] Holmstrup P, Axell T. Classification and clinical manifestations of oral yeast infections. Acta Odontol Scand 1990;48:57–9.

[41] Fotos PG, Vincent SD, Hellstein JW. Oral candidosis: clinical, historical, and therapeutic features of 100 cases. Oral Surg Oral Med Oral Pathol 1992;74:41–9.

[42] Brown R, Krakow AM. Median rhomboid glossitis and a "kissing" lesion of the palate. Oral Surg Oral Med Oral Pathol Oral Radiol Endod 1996;82(5):472–3.

[43] Elzay RP. Traumatic ulcerative granuloma with stromal eosinophilia (Riga-Fede's disease and traumatic eosinophilic granuloma). Oral Surg Oral Med Oral Pathol 1983;55(5): 497–506.

[44] Damm DD, Curran A, White DK, et al. Leukoplakia of the maxillary vestibule—an association with Viadent? Oral Surg Oral Med Oral Pathol Oral Radiol Endod 1999;87(1): 61–6.

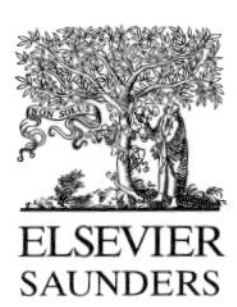

ELSEVIER
SAUNDERS

Otolaryngol Clin N Am
38 (2005) 37–46

OTOLARYNGOLOGIC
CLINICS
OF NORTH AMERICA

# Management of the Clinically Negative Neck in Early Squamous Cell Carcinoma of the Oral Cavity

Scharukh Jalisi, MD

*Department of Otolaryngology-Head and Neck Surgery,
Vanderbilt University Medical Center, S-2100 Medical Center North,
Nashville, TN 37232, USA*

## Epidemiology

Oral cavity squamous cell carcinoma is the sixth leading cause of cancer worldwide [1]. It accounts for 0.6% to 5% of all cancers in Europe, United States, and Australia, respectively, but up to 45% of cancers in India [2]. It mostly affects males, but its incidence is growing among females. It usually occurs in the seventh decade of life. The most common causative factors associated with squamous cell carcinoma of the oral cavity are alcohol and tobacco abuse. Betel nut and tobacco chewing are responsible for the high incidence in the Indian subcontinent.

## Background

The most important prognostic factor in the management of oral squamous cell carcinoma is the status of the cervical lymph nodes [3]. The presence of metastasis to cervical lymph nodes can reduce the cure rate by 50%. Historically the management of the clinically negative (N0) neck has been controversial. Since its description in 1906 by Crile [4] and its routine use by Martin [5], radical neck dissection was the main therapy for any cervical lymph node metastases from head and neck squamous cell carcinoma (HNSCC). The routine use of this operation was questioned and then modified by Bocca et al [6] and Byers [7], especially in patients with limited neck disease and those with clinically negative necks.

*E-mail address:* scharukh.jalisi@vanderbilt.edu

Currently the treatment dilemma that most head and neck oncology surgeons face is the treatment of the N0 neck in oral cavity squamous cell carcinoma. Three treatment options are available:

Observation with therapeutic neck dissection once regional metastases become apparent
Elective neck irradiation
Elective neck dissection

These multiple treatment options, along with different treatment modalities available for the primary cancer, make the neck treatment of early-stage oral cavity squamous cell carcinoma controversial.

## Anatomy

The oral cavity extends from the skin-vermillion junction of the lips to the junction of the hard and soft palate superiorly and to the line of the circumvallate papillae inferiorly. The subsites are [8]

Mucosal lip
Buccal mucosa
Lower alveolar ridge
Upper alveolar ridge
Retromolar trigone
Floor of the mouth
Hard palate
Anterior two thirds of the tongue (oral tongue)

## Management issues and options

Some of the questions that arise when treating an N0 neck in squamous cell carcinoma of the oral cavity are

Is there any noninvasive or invasive modality to assist in diagnosing cervical lymph node metastasis?
Should the neck be treated now or observed?
Are there prognostic factors that can guide decisions on whether or not to treat the neck?
What modality should be used to treat the neck?
Is there an optimal surgical approach to treat the neck?

### Diagnostic modalities

Ideally, the decision about treatment of an N0 neck would be simplified if there were a highly accurate, noninvasive diagnostic modality that could identify metastatic lymph nodes. Studies have shown that the sensitivity, specificity, and accuracy of detection of neck metastases by clinical examination are 70%, 65%, and 68%, respectively. Stuckensen et al [9] compared the usefulness of PET with ultrasound, CT, and MRI in detecting lymph node metastases. Ultrasound had the highest sensitivity (84%), and PET had the highest specificity (82%) among these modalities. Hence, it was concluded that noninvasive diagnostic modalities were not as accurate as histologic sectioning of lymph nodes. Other studies have shown that the detection rate of cervical adenopathy increases from 75% with physical examination alone to 91% when physical examination is combined with CT [10]. Compounding this problem, approximately 8% to 10% of oral and oropharyngeal squamous cell carcinomas have micrometastases to the cervical lymph nodes. These micrometastases can be only 3 mm to 6 mm in diameter, making them pathologically negative during preoperative work-up using current criteria [11–13].

In of oral cavity squamous carcinoma, invasive diagnostic modalities to assess lymph node metastasis include a staging neck dissection (ie, supraomohyoid neck dissection [SOHND]). Davidson et al [14] estimated the accuracy of SOHND in detecting regional metastases to be 98% with a sensitivity of 95% and specificity of 100%, making it currently the best modality for detecting cervical metastases.

*Prognostic factors*

There is voluminous literature discussing different factors that effect prognosis in oral cavity carcinoma. The key factors are presented here.

*Tumor size*

Several studies have shown that increasing tumor size leads to decreased survival. The 5-year survival rates for oral cavity squamous cell carcinoma are 91% for T1 disease, 63% for T2 disease, and 60% for T3 disease. In addition a study by Tytor et al [2] involving 176 patients with oral cavity carcinoma showed that the rate of cervical lymph node metastasis was 14% in patients with T1 tumors, 37% in patients with T2 tumors, and 57% in patients tumors greater than 4 cm in diameter. On the other hand, reports by Rasgon [15] and Byers et al [16] did not show this correlation between the T-stage and cervical node metastasis.

*Perineural invasion and intralymphatic tumor emboli*

Perineural invasion is defined as tumor invasion of the perineural sheath or epineurium. Brown et al [17] demonstrated that regional metastatic disease developed in 71% of N0 patients who had perineural invasion versus 36% of N0 patients who did not have perineural invasion. This study also showed that in the presence of perineural invasion 2-year survival decreased from 82% to 52%. Lydiatt et al [18], in a study of 156 patients with stage I and II tongue cancer, found that local control rate at 5 years was 38% in patients with perineural invasion, versus 78% in patients without perineural invasion. Hence perineural invasion has been associated with decreased survival and with increased local recurrence necessitating more aggressive therapy.

Similarly, 88% of the patients who had intralymphatic tumor emboli in the N0 neck developed regional disease, versus 38% of patients who did not have such emboli [17].

*DNA ploidy*

In one study, bone invasion occurred in 68% of patients with DNA nondiploid tumors, versus 22% of patients with DNA diploid tumors [2]. Nodal metastases occurred in 54% of DNA nondiploid and 19% of DNA diploid tumors. Rasgon [15] and Mendelson et al [19] showed a relationship between differentiation grade and the rate of cervical lymph node metastases. Hence, discussion of the DNA diploid state and grade of the tumor with a pathologist is important in treatment planning.

*Tumor thickness*

In recent years the relationship of occult cervical lymph node metastasis with thickness of the tumor has been widely investigated.

Fukano et al [20] showed in 34 patients that cervical metastasis increased from 5.9% for tongue carcinomas less than 5 mm thick to 64.7% for tongue carcinomas more than 5 mm thick. Brown et al [17] noted that 38% of patients with tumor thickness less than 3 mm developed regional disease, compared with 41% of patients with tumor thickness of 3 mm to 7 mm and with 55% of patients with tumor thickness greater than 7 mm. He also showed that increasing tumor thickness is associated with greater perineural invasion. Fakih et al [21] noted that in T1 and T2 squamous cell carcinoma of the oral tongue a thickness greater than 4 mm is associated with a greater risk of neck relapse. Another study noted that the rate of rate of occult cervical metastases increased from 7% to 30% when the thickness of the tumor was greater than or equal to 4 mm [22].

A study of 156 patients with stage I and II squamous cell carcinoma lesion of the floor of mouth demonstrated that cervical metastasis occurred in 2% of cases with thickness less than 1.5 mm, in 33% of cases with thickness of 1.6 mm to 3.5 mm, and in 60% of cases with thickness greater than 3.6 mm. The investigators concluded that elective neck dissection (END) should be undertaken in floor of mouth squamous cell carcinomas more than 1.5 mm thick [23].

Tumor thickness has also been shown to correlate with survival in several studies. In one such study [17, the 2-year survival rate was 94% for tumors less than 3 mm thick, was 69% for tumors greater than 3 mm but less than 7 mm thick, and decreased to 58% for tumors more than 7 mm thick. Similarly Urist et al [24] had shown improved survival in buccal cancer patients when thickness is less than 6 mm.

*Extracapsular spread*

The presence of extracapsular spread (ECS) further reduces survival. In a retrospective review by Alvi and Johnson [25] of N0 neck dissection specimens, the occult metastatic rate was 34%, and ECS was noted in 49% of these specimens. In the presence of ECS the 2-year survival decreased from 47% to 31%. The authors recommended adjuvant therapy in the presence of ECS.

Hence, multiple factors that can affect the rate of cervical metastasis and survival from oral cavity cancer. It is important for the head and neck oncologic surgeon to be familiar with these factors to be able to provide patients the best counsel about the appropriate treatment modalities.

## Observation versus elective neck treatment

There is great controversy regarding the optimal therapy for clinically negative necks. The proponents of observation cite the morbidity of END as a reason to observe. Another argument for close observation is that with close follow-up, any cervical metastasis can be detected early and then treated with adequate therapy. Moreover the occult metastatic rate to the neck from oral cavity cancer is 34% [3]. Hence, it is argued that nearly two thirds of the patients would be exposed to the morbidity of a neck dissection unnecessarily.

On the other hand Weiss et al [26] created a decision-tree analysis and concluded that observation is the preferred option when the probability of occult metastasis is less than 20% and elective neck treatment (irradiation or dissection) is preferred if the probability of occult metastasis is greater than 20%. In squamous cell carcinoma of the oral cavity the sites with a less than 20% occult metastatic rate to the neck are T1/T2 lip carcinomas, T1/T2 oral tongue carcinomas that are less than 4 mm thick, and T1/T2 floor of mouth cancers less than or equal to 1.5 mm thick.

The proponents of surgical intervention also note that removal of lymph nodes can be used as a staging procedure. If there is presence of extracapsular spread, the patient can be upstaged and receive more aggressive therapy early on rather than later when survival may be adversely affected. Andersen et al [27] demonstrated that 77% of patients with clinically N0 necks at initial observation had pathologically adverse findings at the time of neck dissection. Furthermore 49% of these patients had ECS, a poor prognostic factor. Hence, they argued for elective neck treatment (irradiation or neck dissection) in patients with N0 necks.

Another study comparing glossectomy and neck observation versus glossectomy and neck dissection for T1 and T2 squamous cell carcinoma of the oral tongue concluded that survival in the observation group was 33%, compared with 55% in the neck dissection group, and that locoregional control increased from 50% to 91% when neck dissection was performed. Again, the rate of ECS in this study was noted to be 58% in patients who were observed [18]. A similar study comparing 5-year survival in T1/T2 N0 squamous cell carcinoma of the oral tongue found that the survival rate decreased from 80.5% to 44.8% when a delayed neck dissection was performed [28]. Kligerman et al [22] had shown that in early carcinoma of the oral cavity the addition of a SOHND increased 3-year survival from 49% to 72%.

Wendt et al [29] reported that, in 103 patients with T1 and T2 N0 squamous cell carcinoma of the oral tongue, neck recurrence occurred in 44% patients who received no radiation treatment to the neck, in 27% of those receiving less than 40 Gy to the neck, and in 11% of patients receiving more than 40 Gy to the neck.

In summary, although the decision to observe or treat the N0 neck is left to the choice of the patient and the head and neck oncologist, in oral cavity carcinoma the only clinically N0 necks for which observation is appropriate are those associated with T1/T2 lip carcinomas, T1/T2 oral tongue carcinomas that are less than 4 mm thick, and T1/T2 floor of mouth cancers less than or equal to 1.5 mm thick.

## Elective neck dissection versus elective neck irradiation

Once the decision to treat the N0 neck has been made, there are two possible treatment modalities. The question then arises whether to irradiate the neck or to perform a surgical lymphadenectomy.

Mendenhall et al [30] showed that elective neck irradiation (ENI) reduced the neck failure rate in patients with controlled primary tumors and N0 necks from 18% to 1.9%. The dose of radiation varied from 50 Gy to 75 Gy in the upper neck and from 40 Gy to 50 Gy in the lower neck. Another study reported that ENI provided a 95% control rate for neck recurrences compared with 38% without ENI in T1 N0 squamous cell carcinoma of the oral tongue [31]. Hence, the neck recurrence rate can be extrapolated to be 5%, which is comparable to the 4% to 7% recurrence rate noted in electiveneck dissection [32]. At the University of Virginia the preference is ENI for N0 necks [33].

The modality that is chosen to treat the primary cancer may also help in formulating a decision as to how to treat the neck. If primary radiation therapy is used, ENI can be performed. If the neck is going to be entered to remove the primary tumor, an END can be performed. Obviously, the risks of ENI and END need to be considered on an individual basis for each patient.

The argument for END is that it can be used as a staging procedure and hence help in determining the need for any future therapy. Also, the risk of a second primary tumor in treated cancers of the oral cavity is 4% to 6% per year [34]. Hence, using ENI in patients with early squamous cell carcinoma of the oral cavity may exhaust the use of radiation therapy as a treatment in the event of a future head and neck cancer. Other morbidities associated with ENI are xerostomia, dysphagia, greater oral passage time after radiation therapy, mucositis, pain, poor wound healing, increased complications if salvage surgery is performed, longer duration of therapy (up to

6 weeks), cost of travel, and time away from work. In a series of 85 patients treated for T1 and T2 N0 squamous cell carcinoma of the oral tongue, Al-Rajhi et al [35] demonstrated that the rate of neck recurrence was 35% in patients who were observed, 39% in patients who received ENI, and 19% in patients who received END. These investigators concluded that END is the modality of choice for treatment of the N0 neck. They used ENI with a total dose of 45 to 50 Gy, however, and showed no survival difference between the three groups.

Chow et al [36] demonstrated that after 5-year follow-up there was no statistical difference between ENI and END in regard to neck recurrence for cancers of the oral cavity, oropharynx, and larynx.

In summary the literature provides no clear-cut recommendation for using ENI or END to treat N0 necks. The most important factors in guiding this decision should be the patient's informed decision, physician and institution experience, risk of second primary occurrence in the future, and the modality chosen to treat the primary cancer.

## Elective neck dissection—which surgery should be performed?

The lymph nodes at highest risk of occult metastases from oral cavity cancers are those at levels I, II, and III [3]. The metastatic rates to these sites are 58% (level I), 51% (level II), 26% (level III), 9% (level IV), and 2% (level V). There has been a long-lasting debate about the relative efficacy of SOHND and that of a classic radical neck dissection. Several studies have shown that there is no statistically significant difference in locoregional recurrence between a selective neck dissection and a radical neck dissection [32]. Byers et al [37] noted a skip metastasis rate of 15% to level IV in squamous cell carcinoma of the oral tongue and advocated that dissection of level IV should be included in a selective neck dissection. More recently it has been demonstrated that level IV need be dissected only if there are suspicious nodes in level II or III [38]. In conclusion, there is voluminous literature supporting the use of selective neck dissection for surgical treatment of N0 necks in oral cavity carcinoma. This procedure has relatively low morbidity when compared with the classic radical neck dissection.

## Combined-modality treatment

In several situations postoperative radiation or salvage surgery is necessary. Several authors [18,32,39] and the Head and Neck Society [40] guidelines recommend the use of postoperative radiation therapy when there are perineural, intravascular, and intralymphatic tumor spread, positive microscopic margins, more than two histologically positive lymph nodes, multiple positive lymph nodes, extracapsular spread, and DNA nondiploid tumors.

## Management of the contralateral N0 neck

Another issue of concern is the treatment of the contralateral N0 neck. A study showed that there was a 14% incidence of involvement of contra-lateral neck nodes regardless of tumor stage. The Head and Neck Society recommends the treatment of the contralateral nodes if the primary oral cavity cancer is midline, bilateral, along the tip of the tongue, or approaches or crosses the midline.

## Future directions

The difficult choices that need to be made and discussed with patients would be easier if there were a noninvasive technology that could correctly identify metastatic lymph nodes in a N0 neck. Currently proton magnetic resonance spectroscopy is being investigated for this purpose [41,42].

In squamous cell carcinoma, sentinel node biopsy has been used with mixed results. It has been used in melanoma of the head and neck. Koch et al [43] concluded the difficulty with this method for oral cavity squamous cell carcinoma. Alex et al [44], on the other hand, showed that in eight cases sentinel node biopsy correctly identified the metastatic node in every case. Obviously more research, including large, prospective, randomized studies, is needed before this modality will be widely accepted in this realm.

## Summary

1. Management of the N0 neck in squamous cell carcinoma of the oral cavity is controversial.
2. The N0 neck should be treated if the risk of occult metastasis is greater than 20%.
3. Sites where the neck can be observed are T1/T2 squamous lip carcinomas, T1/T2 oral tongue squamous carcinomas that are less than 4 mm thick, and T1/T2 squamous floor of mouth cancers less than or equal to 1.5 mm thick.
4. ENI and END seem to have comparable control rates (except in a study by Al- Rajhi [34]).
5. Ultimately the decision to treat the neck and the modality used depend on the patient's preference, physician and institution experience, the risk of a second primary cancer in the future, and the modality used to treat the primary cancer.
6. Development of future technologies and large, randomized, prospective trials of these technologies will shape the future of this treatment dilemma.

## References

[1] Landis SH, Murray T, Bolden S, et al. Cancer statistics, 1999. CA Cancer J Clin 1999;49: 8–31.

[2] Tytor M, Olofsson J. Prognostic factors in oral cavity carcinoma. Acta Otolaryngol 1992;(Suppl 492):75–8.

[3] Shah JP. Patterns of cervical lymph node metastasis from squamous carcinomas of the upper aerodigestive tract. Am J Surg 1990;160:405–9.

[4] Crile GW. Excision of cancer of the head and neck. JAMA 1906;47:1780–6.

[5] Martin H, DelValle B, Ehrich H, et al. Neck dissection. Cancer 1951;4:441–99.

[6] Bocca E, Pignatarao O, Oidini C, et al. Functional neck dissection: an evaluation of 853 cases. Laryngoscope 1984;94:942–5.

[7] Byers RM. Modified neck dissection: a study of 967 cases from 1970 to 1980. Am J Surg 1985; 150:414–21.

[8] Greene FL, Page DL, Fleming ID, et al. Lip and oral cavity. In: American Joint Committee on Cancer cancer staging manual. 6th edition. New York: Springer; 2002. p. 23–32.

[9] Stuckensen T, Kovacs AF, Adams S, et al. Staging of the neck in patients with oral cavity squamous cell carcinomas: a prospective comparison of PET, ultrasound, CT and MRI. J Craniomaxillofac Surg 2000;28:319–24.

[10] Merritt RM, Williams MF, James TH, et al. Detection of cervical metastasis. A meta-analysis comparing computed tomography with physical examination. Arch Otolaryngol Head Neck Surg 1997;123:149–52.

[11] Ambrosch P, Kron M, Fischer G, et al. Micrometastases in carcinoma of the upper aerodigestive tract: detection, risk of metastasizing, and prognostic value of depth of invasion. Head Neck 1995;17(6):473–9.

[12] Van den Brekel MW, Stel HV, van der Valk P, et al. Micrometastases from squamous cell carcinoma in neck dissection specimens. Eur Arch Otorhinolaryngol 1992;249(6):349–53.

[13] Barrera JE, Miller ME, Said S, et al. Detection of occult cervical micrometastases in patients with head and neck squamous cell cancer. Laryngoscope 2003;113(5):892–6.

[14] Davidson J, Biem J, Detsky A. The clinically negative neck in patients with early oral cavity carcinoma: a decision analysis approach to management. J Otolaryngol 1995;24: 323–9.

[15] Rasgon B, Cruz R, Hilsinger R. Relation of lymph node metastasis to histopathologic appearance in oral cavity and oropharyngeal carcinoma: a case series and literature review. Laryngoscope 1989;99:1103–10.

[16] Byers RM, Wolf PF, Ballantyne AJ. Rationale for elective modified neck dissection. Head Neck 1988;10:160–7.

[17] Brown B, Barnes L, Mazariegos J, et al. Prognostic factors in mobile tongue and floor of mouth carcinoma. Cancer 1989;64:1195–202.

[18] Lydiatt DD, Robbins KT, Byers RM, et al. Treatment of stage I and II oral tongue cancer. Head Neck 1993;15:308–12.

[19] Mendelson BC, Woods JE, Beahrs OH. Neck dissection in the treatment of carcinoma of the anterior two-thirds of the tongue. Surgery, Gynecology & Obstetrics 1976;143:75–80.

[20] Fukano H, Matsuura H, Hasegawa Y, et al. Depth of invasion as a predictive factor for cervical lymph node metastasis in tongue carcinoma. Head Neck 1997;19:205–10.

[21] Fakih AR, Rao RS, Borges AM, et al. Elective versus therapeutic neck dissection in early carcinoma of the oral tongue. Am J Surg 1989;158:308–13.

[22] Kligerman J, Lima RA, Soares JR, et al. Supraomohyoid neck dissection in the treatment of T1/T2 squamous cell carcinoma of oral cavity. Am J Surg 1994;168:391–4.

[23] Mohit-Tabatabai MA, Sobel HJ, Rush BF, et al. Relation of thickness of floor of mouth stage I and II cancers to regional metastasis. Am J Surg 1986;152:351–3.

[24] Urist MM, O'Brien CJ, Soong SJ, et al. Squamous cell carcinoma of the buccal mucosa: analysis of prognostic factors. Am J Surg 1987;154:411–4.

[25] Alvi A, Johnson JT. Extracapsular spread in the clinically negative neck (N0): implications and outcome. Otolaryngol Head Neck Surg 1996;114:65–70.

[26] Weiss MH, Harrison LB, Isaacs RS. Use of decision analysis in planning a management strategy for the stage N0 neck. Arch Otolaryngol Head Neck Surg 1994;120:699–702.

[27] Andersen PE, Cambronero E, Shaha AR, et al. The extent of neck disease after regional failure during observation of the N0 neck. Am J Surg 1996;172:689–91.

[28] Haddadin KJ, Soutar DS, Oliver RJ, et al. Improved survival for patients with clinically T1/T2, N0 tongue tumors undergoing a prophylactic neck dissection. Head Neck 1999;21(6): 517–25.

[29] Wendt CD, Peters LJ, Delclos L, et al. Primary radiotherapy in the treatment of stage I and II oral tongue cancers: importance of the proportion of therapy delivered with interstitial therapy. Int J Radiat Oncol Biol Phys 1990;18:1287–92.

[30] Mendenhall WM, Million RR, Cassisi NJ. Elective neck irradiation in squamous cell carcinoma of the head and neck. Head Neck Surg 1980;3(1):15–20.

[31] Spaulding CA, Korb LJ, Constable WC, et al. The influence of extent of neck treatment upon control of cervical lymphadenopathy in cancers of the oral tongue. Int J Radiat Oncol Biol Phys 1991;21:577–81.

[32] Pitman KT, Johnson JT, Myers EN. Effectiveness of selective neck dissection for management of the clinically negative neck. Arch Otolaryngol Head Neck Surg 1997;123:917–22.

[33] Levine PA, Hood JR. Neoplasms of the oral cavity. In: Bailey BJ, Calhoun KH, Healy GB, et al, editors. Head and neck surgery-otolaryngology. 3rd edition. Philadelphia: Lippincott Williams and Wilkins; 2001. p. 1311–25.

[34] Wolfensberger M, Zbaeren P, Dulguerov P, et al. Surgical treatment of early oral carcinoma—results of a prospective controlled multicenter study. Head Neck 2001;23: 525–30.

[35] Al-Rajhi N, Khafaga Y, El-Husseiny J, et al. Early stage carcinoma of oral tongue: prognostic factors for local control and survival. Oral Oncol 2000;36:508–14.

[36] Chow JM, Levin BC, Krivit JS, et al. Radiotherapy or surgery for subclinical cervical node metastases. Arch Otolaryngol Head Neck Surg 1989;115:981–4.

[37] Byers RM, Weber RS, Andrews T, et al. Frequency and therapeutic implications of 'skip metastases' in the neck from squamous carcinoma of the oral tongue. Head Neck 1997;19: 14–9.

[38] Khafif A, Lopez-Garza JR, Medina JE. Is dissection of level IV necessary in patients with T1–3 N0 tongue cancer? Laryngoscope 2001;111:1088–90.

[39] Myers EN, Cunningham MJ. Treatments of choice for early carcinoma of the oral cavity. Oncology 1988;2:18–24.

[40] American Head and Neck Society. Tumors of the upper aerodigestive tract: oral cavity. Available at: www.headandneckcancer.org/clinicalresources/docs/oralcavity.php. Accessed November 2, 2004.

[41] Star-Lack JM, Adalsteinsson E, Adam ME, et al. In vivo 1H MR spectroscopy of human head and neck lymph node metastasis and comparison with oxygen tension measurements. Am J Neuroradiol 2000;21:183–93.

[42] Pitman KT, Dean R. Management of the clinically negative (N0) neck. Curr Oncol Rep 2002;4(1):81–6.

[43] Koch W, Choti M, Civelek A, et al. Gamma probe-directed biopsy of the sentinel node in oral squamous cell carcinoma. Arch Otolaryngol 1998;27:342–7.

[44] Alex JC, Sasaki CT, Krag DN, et al. Sentinel lymph node radiolocalization in head and neck squamous cell carcinoma. Laryngoscopy 2000;110:198–203.

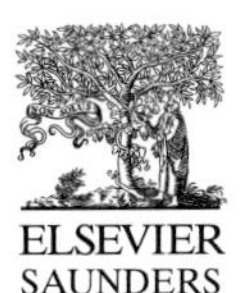

ELSEVIER
SAUNDERS

Otolaryngol Clin N Am
38 (2005) 47–57

OTOLARYNGOLOGIC
CLINICS
OF NORTH AMERICA

# Advanced Laryngeal Carcinoma: Surgical and Non-surgical Management Options

M. Jalisi, FCPS, FRCS[a,b], Scharukh Jalisi, MD[c,*]

[a]Department of Otolaryngology, College of Physicians and Surgeons, Pakistan
[b]J. J. Hospital, Karachi, Pakistan
[c]Department of Otolaryngology-Head and Neck Surgery,
Vanderbilt University Medical Center, Nashville, TN 37232, USA

In this article advanced laryngeal carcinoma is defined as clinical stage III and clinical stage IV malignant tumors arising from the laryngeal epithelium. This advanced stage depends on tumor size, presence of neck disease, or both (Box 1) [1].

A further elaboration of the definition would include the term "anaplastic or undifferentiated" in the overall description. According to one study, these tumors account for 46.03% of all squamous cell cancers that occur in the larynx [2] and therefore 0.46% of all malignancies in humans [3].

## Classification

Classification is fundamental for the understanding of epidemiology, for therapeutic decision-making, and for preemptive prognosis. Although Broder's grading [4] is still mentioned in histopathologic reports, the TNM classification [1] as accepted by the International Union against Cancer (UICC) and the American Joint Committee on Cancer (AJCC) in 1978 is more pertinent and therefore is widely followed. TNM staging considers anatomic distribution and T-staging together with nodal status and presence or absence of distant metastasis.

The larynx is divided into three regions for studying anatomic distribution of laryngeal carcinoma: supraglottic, glottic, and subglottic. The glottic region extends from the floor of the ventricles to the undersurface of

---

* Corresponding author. S2100 Medical Center North, 47 Chaffee Road, Nashville, TN 37232.

*E-mail address:* scharukh@hotmail.com (S. Jalisi).

---

**Box 1. Staging of advanced laryngeal tumors according to the American Joint Committee on Cancer Staging [1]**

*Stage III tumors*
 T1, N1, M0
 T2, N1, M0
 T3 N0 M0
 T3, N1, M0

*Stage IV tumors*
 Stage 4 A
 T4 N0 M0
 T4, N1, M0
 Any T, N2, M0
 Stage 4 B
 Any T, N3, M0
 Stage 4 C
 Any T, Any N, M1

---

the true vocal folds. The supraglottic and subglottic regions lie above and below the glottis, respectively. The supraglottic region is further divided into an upper epilarynx and a lower supraglottis. The epilarynx is comprised of the suprahyoid epiglottis, the right and left arytenoids, and the two aryepiglottic folds. The supraglottis consists of the infrahyoid epiglottis, the laryngeal ventricles, and the two false vocal cords. The distribution of laryngeal carcinoma among these subsites is 76% in the glottic area, 19% in the supraglottic area, and 5% in the subglottic region. The most common site for carcinoma to develop is the vocal cords (73%) [3]. The aryepiglottic folds and false vocal cords follow suit with 7% and 5%, respectively. The anterior commissure is involved in 2% of cases and is perhaps the most dangerous area in which cancer occurs, followed by the subglottic area. At the anterior commissure a thin fibrous tendon connects a very thin laryngeal submucosa directly with the thyroid cartilage. The intervening tissue barrier consisting of Reinke's membrane and the conus elasticus is missing. As a result even a T1 neoplasm involving this area can frequently invade the cartilaginous laryngeal frame in the midline [5] and become a T4 tumor. The subglottic area is not easily visible to the examining eye. Also, subglottic tumors present late, usually after the vocal cords are involved, and metastasize to rather inaccessible mediastinal lymph glands.

In 1954 the UICC began trying to formalize a TNM-based classification of malignant tumors, including those that affect the larynx. Not until 1978 was a consensus developed with the AJCC, and a classification of laryngeal cancers was finalized. This classification has since been updated [1]. The main denominators in this classification are the letters *T*, which stands for tumor size, $N$, which denotes regional lymph node secondary tumors, and $M$, which indicates tumor metastasis to distant areas below the clavicle or above the skull base. Further details of the classification can be found in the American Joint Committee on Cancer *Staging Manual* (sixth edition) [1].

## Treatment

During the last 10 years, there has been a complete reconsideration of the options for treating advanced laryngeal cancer. At one time the only options considered were radiotherapy or surgery [6]. Surgery was considered efficient but mutilating [7]. Billroth of Vienna did the first total laryngectomy for cancer in 1873, but the operation was not widely adopted until the next century because it was mutilating and fraught with complications [8]. Undoubtedly it gave efficient local site control, but it resulted in the loss of laryngeal functions and airway integrity [9]. Radiotherapy preserved the larynx, but it required mutilating laryngeal surgery for salvage. Later came the era of surgery in combination with postoperative radiotherapy. Often concurrent or induction chemotherapy was added to this regimen to improve the results [10]. This approach gave most patients a longer disease-free survival, but the loss of laryngeal functions still remained. As a result a new paradigm was developed in which organ preservation replaced all other considerations. To preserve function, surgical techniques aimed at conserving functionally important tissues were developed. These new operations, usually in combination with radiotherapy or chemotherapy, could obtain the desired oncologic and functional outcomes in terms of speech, swallowing, respiration, and airway integrity [12]. At the same time organ-preserving chemotherapy and radiotherapy protocols were created.

The present scenario is therefore encouraging. Palliative treatment is given to the approximately 11% of patients who initially present with distant metastases. For the remaining 89%, a large spectrum of new techniques [11] offers disease clearance, functional preservation, and, in combination with radiotherapy and chemotherapy, longer disease-free survival. The standard surgical treatment as practiced today consists of induction chemotherapy followed by conservation surgery and postoperative radiotherapy.

## Palliation

Palliation aims at suppressing the cancer and its symptoms without any real intent to cure. It is indicated for terminal cases and for patients who refuse other forms of treatment. In advanced laryngeal cancer, palliation consists of

1. Pharmacologic treatment of pain. In advanced laryngeal cancer, some patients complain of pain. This pain is usually referred to the ipsilateral ear but may also be felt elsewhere in the head and neck. In most patients

therapeutic doses of narcotics or nonsteroidal anti-inflammatory drugs given either by mouth or parenterally are effective. Sometimes, a supplement of some sedative drug (eg, diazepam) may also be required. Rarely, pain relief requires more intense measures such as removal of larynx, removal of nodal metastases in the neck, radiotherapy, and chemotherapy.

2. Tracheostomy. Tracheostomy is indicated to obviate dyspnea, which may be distressing in some cases. Another reason for tracheostomy is pulmonary toilet. With a massive growth in the larynx, the patient may not be able to cough and therefore needs assistance to clear secretions.

3. Radiotherapy. Radiotherapy for palliation is time honored. It is given locally, focusing on the area of symptoms. Doses are given in smaller fractions and shorter courses unless they are tolerated well.

4. Chemotherapy. Chemotherapy is also used for palliation. Usually a combination of chemotherapeutic agents (eg, cisplatin plus 5-fluorouracil or methotrexate plus bleomycin) is used. The expected outcomes include regression of lesions and relief of symptoms. Significant side effects may occur.

## Curative treatment

Organ preservation is the mainstay of modern curative treatment. It encompasses all modalities and options that satisfy this principle and preserve laryngeal functions. As outlined in Box 2, these techniques include radiotherapy, chemotherapy, and surgical approaches that have been refined during the last decade or so.

Vertical partial laryngeal resections are performed through a laryngofissure. Epiglottectomy and supraglottic partial laryngectomy (SGPL) are done through an anterior pharyngotomy. More recently this type of conservation surgery has also been performed through transoral laser surgery [12]. Supracricoid partial laryngectomy (SCPL) entails resection of the thyroid cartilage, pre-epiglottic space, paraglottic space, and one of the two arytenoids. The epiglottis may or may not be resected. The hyoid bone, cricoid cartilage, and the remaining arytenoid are preserved. A crico-hyoidopexy or crico-hyoidoepiglottopexy is used for closure of the larynx.

Indications for a SCPL are [21]

1. Selected T1 supraglottic tumors involving the infrahyoid epiglottis or ventricle
2. Selected T2 transglottic and supraglottic tumors
3. Selected T3 transglottic and supraglottic tumors with true vocal cord fixation or limited pre-epiglottic space invasion, without arytenoid involvement
4. Selected T4 transglottic and supraglottic tumors with limited invasion of the thyroid ala without extension through the outer perichondrium

---

**Box 2. Curative treatment for laryngeal carcinoma**

1. Vertical partial resection
   Cordectomy
   Frontal partial laryngectomy
   Lateral partial laryngectomy
   Frontolateral partial laryngectomy
2. Horizontal partial resection
   Epiglottectomy
   Supraglottic partial laryngectomy
3. More extensive partial resection
   Supracricoid partial laryngectomy
   Near-total laryngectomy

---

Contraindications for SCPL are [21]

1. Arytenoid cartilage fixation. Because of cricoarytenoid joint fixation, the cricoid cartilage cannot be spared.
2. Infraglottic extension of tumor more than 10 mm anteriorly or 5 mm posterolaterally
3. Extensive invasion of the pre-epiglottic space
4. Tumor extending to the hyoid bone superiorly or the cricoid cartilage inferiorly. Reconstruction will be almost impossible if these structures are removed.
5. Extralaryngeal tumor spread

Total laryngectomy in conjunction with procedures such as tracheoesophageal puncture is now restricted to T4 lesions not amenable to SCPL, to radiation failures, and to salvage after failed conservation surgery. Radiotherapy is no longer a primary modality in the treatment of laryngeal cancer except for T1a and T1b lesions of glottic area and for a well-differentiated carcinoma situated in the middle of a mobile vocal cord (T1a). The same is true for chemotherapy. These two modalities are now used in conjunction with surgery and for palliation purposes in cases with distant metastases (M1). Whereas chemotherapy sensitizes the tissues to the action of radiotherapy, postoperative radiotherapy improves the prognosis in cases treated with surgery.

Options for surgical treatment of advanced laryngeal tumors in cases other than those with distant metastases (M1) are summarized here.

*Supraglottic carcinoma*

*T3 N0 disease*
In treating T3 N0 disease, there is a choice between SGPL and SCPL. Cases with extension into pre-epiglottic space or involvement of the anterior

commissure, the glottis, and the hypopharynx are treated with SCPL, provided at least one arytenoid cartilage is disease free with clear margins. All other cases are dealt with SGCL. In both groups induction chemotherapy and postoperative radiotherapy are given to improve results.

### T4 N0 disease

T4 N0 cases may be treated with SCPL (see indications listed previously) that gives efficient disease clearance along with preservation of laryngeal functions and integrity of airway. If both arytenoids are involved or the cricoid cartilage is infiltrated, SCPL is contraindicated. In that case total laryngectomy with some speech reconstruction procedure is undertaken. In both groups induction chemotherapy and postoperative radiotherapy are given to improve results.

## Glottic carcinoma

### T3 N0 disease

T3 N0 cases are treated with frontolateral partial laryngectomy, which is also called "hemilaryngectomy." When the paraglottic space, anterior commissure, and thyroid cartilage are involved, SCPL is performed. If there is any contraindication to SCPL or if salvage surgery for recurrence needs to be performed, total laryngectomy with some speech reconstruction procedure is performed. In all groups induction chemotherapy and postoperative radiotherapy are given to improve results.

### T4 N0 disease

The treatment for T4 N0 cases is the same as for the T4 N0 supraglottic carcinoma, that is, SCPL. If there is any contraindication to this procedure, total laryngectomy is done along with tracheoesophageal puncture or some other speech reconstruction procedure. In both groups induction chemotherapy and postoperative radiotherapy are given to improve results.

## Subglottic carcinoma

Subglottic tumors are not easily visible on laryngoscopy. Also, they present late and metastasize to mediastinal lymph glands that are not palpable on routine clinical examination. Furthermore, the subglottis abuts the cricoid cartilage, which therefore is involved in many cases. Therefore SCPL is contraindicated in such patients. Induction chemotherapy followed by total laryngectomy and postoperative radiotherapy is the treatment of choice Because of the possibility of mediastinal spread, postoperative radiation should cover both the lower neck and mediastinum [13,14].

Induction chemotherapy before surgery has been suggested because of the presence of an intact blood supply, a more responsive cell mass, the elimination of micrometastases, and possibility of tumor regression. Because of synergism, various drug combinations (eg, cisplatin plus 5-fluorouracil or methotrexate plus bleomycin) are preferred over single agents. The drugs administered should have the least toxicity with demonstrable response against the cancer. Furthermore, results are better if cancer chemotherapeutics are given in short spurts (eg, for 24–36 hours) and intermittent courses (eg, 3–4 weeks) [15].

## Management of neck disease

The risk of occult metastasis is approximately 40% from the supraglottis (which can be bilateral) and 24% from the glottis [22]. According to the clinical guidelines of the American Head and Neck Society [23], in the presence of a N0 neck (no demonstrable secondary tumors in the neck), both the ipsilateral and the contralateral neck need to be addressed either through a selective neck dissection (level II, III, IV) or by elective neck irradiation, especially in supraglottic cancer. N1 disease may be managed by an ipsilateral selective neck dissection. More aggressive neck dissection may be performed depending on the location of the lymph node. N2-N3 disease generally requires a comprehensive modified radical neck dissection or a radical neck dissection. For supraglottic cancer, bilateral neck treatment is important because of the high likelihood for metastasis in the contralateral neck. Obviously, bilateral neck dissection will be performed for midline lesions. The final decision to treat the neck depends upon the patient's preference, on input from medical and radiation oncology and the head and neck surgeon, and on the modality used to treat the primary cancer.

## Nonsurgical management

Nonsurgical approaches to larynx preservation include radiation alone, neoadjuvant chemotherapy with radiation for responders, or concurrent chemotherapy and radiation therapy [24,25]. These management approaches have been used in response to a shift in paradigm to avoid a total laryngectomy whenever possible. Many patients choose to forgo the chance of cure through a total laryngectomy in return for the superior quality of life afforded by an intact airway and useable voice.

The Veterans Affairs (VA) Laryngeal Cancer Study Group published its results in 1991 [26]. This study randomly assigned 332 patients with stage III or stage IV laryngeal cancer to receive induction chemotherapy with two cycles of cisplatin-fluorouracil followed either by a third cycle and then radiation therapy (in responders) or by total laryngectomy and postoperative radiation (in nonresponders). Patients in the chemoradiation group were treated with salvage laryngectomy when there was a less than 50% reduction in tumor size, posttreatment persistence of tumor, or tumor recurrence. In the chemotherapy group 36% of the patients who did not respond to the chemotherapy were referred for total laryngectomy and postoperative radiation therapy. The estimated 2-year survival in this study was 68% for both the surgery and chemoradiation arms. The larynx was preserved in 64% of patients in the chemoradiation group, and 64% of patients in this group were alive and free of disease at 2 years. Hence, the authors concluded that a positive response to induction chemotherapy may be used as an indication to proceed with radiation therapy instead of surgery. Critics of this study noted that this study did not prove the survival benefit of chemotherapy because there was no arm for treatment by radiation therapy alone [27]. Furthermore neoadjuvant chemotherapy has little proven value except as a radiosensitizer [24].

Follow-up studies to the VA laryngeal study group assessed the functionality of patients treated in the chemoradiation group. This group had better objective speech, and only two patients required a tracheostomy [28,29]. After a 10-year follow-up, however, there was no difference in self-reported assessment of speech and swallowing between the two groups [30]. Other studies have demonstrated significant swallowing dysfunction after chemoradiation [28].

In 2001 Forastiere et al [31] presented preliminary results of the three-arm trial conducted by the National Cancer Institute Cooperative Trials Head and Neck Intergroup (R91-11). In this trial, 547 patients were randomly assigned to one of three arms: induction chemotherapy and radiotherapy (A), concomitant chemoradiotherapy (B), or radiation therapy alone (C). There was no difference in survival in the three groups at 2 years. Laryngectomy-free survival was longer in arm B (66%) than in arm A (58%) or arm C (52%).

In another study [32], 80 patients with stage III and IV laryngeal cancer were assigned to receive either radiation therapy alone or neoadjuvant chemotherapy followed by radiation therapy. The 5-year survival was similar in the two groups (24% for radiation therapy alone versus 31% for combined group). The laryngeal preservation rate was also similar at 62% for the former group and 63% for the latter group. Hence, it was concluded that radiation therapy without neoadjuvant chemotherapy is a viable alternative to treatment of advanced laryngeal carcinoma.

Organ-preservation protocols should be avoided in patients with major pre-epiglottic and paraglottic spread, cartilage destruction, massive subglottic disease, and major soft tissue extension. In such situations consideration should be given to total laryngectomy with postoperative radiation therapy for the best oncologic result [24]. Furthermore organ preservation does not equate with organ function, and patients who have undergone nonsurgical management do have swallowing and vocal quality problems [24,27].

There are several disadvantages to treating patients with nonsurgical chemotherapy and radiation therapy protocols. These disadvantages include the risk of major mucosal necrosis or chondronecrosis in case endolaryngeal biopsies need to be performed for surveillance. Moreover, surgical salvage after tumor persistence or recurrence requires a total laryngectomy and can be complex. The complication rate ranges from 33% to 61% according to some studies [33,34].

## Prognosis

With 73% of carcinomas occurring on the vocal cords, the larynx is perhaps the best place to have a malignancy. The vocal cords are functionally active most of the time and hence the slightest suspicion of functional aberration is detected early. Moreover, they do not have a rich lymphatic network, so the rate of neck metastasis from the glottis is low. Besides, a continuous sheet of connective tissue, Reinke's membrane, surrounds the larynx. The net result of these special attributes is early diagnosis and late spread of cancers occurring here. Therefore prognosis of these tumors is good. A number of controlled clinical trials performed at different centers have demonstrated positive treatment results even in advanced cases. Thus in supraglottic carcinomas recurring after radiotherapy and treated with SGPL, the 5-year survival rate is 70% [7]. Similarly, failures and more advanced T4 supraglottic tumors treated by SCPL or by total laryngectomy when SCPL is contraindicated also have a reasonable prognosis. Radiotherapy failures in T1 and T2 glottic tumors treated with hemilaryngectomy have a 3-year survival rate of 60% [16]. The 5-year survival rate for failures and more extensive T3 and T4 glottic tumors treated with total laryngectomy is 47% [17]. Subglottic cases treated with radical surgery and postoperative radiotherapy have a similar prognosis. Hill and Price [18] reported a 7-year survival rate of 63% in 65 cases of advanced laryngeal cancer that they treated with two cycles of induction chemotherapy followed by surgery and postoperative radiotherapy. Kisch et al [19] reported a 5-year survival rate of 79% in 85 cases of advanced head and neck cancer that they treated with three courses of cisplatin in combination with 5-fluorouracil at monthly intervals followed by surgery and postoperative radiotherapy. Jacob et al [20] treated 462 cases of advanced, recurrent, and metastatic disease (48% of which had metastatic disease) with induction chemotherapy using cisplatin plus bleomycin followed by surgery and postoperative radiotherapy. The major response rate at the end of 2 years was 37%. In summary, when advanced laryngeal cancer is treated with surgery and radiation, the 5-year survival ranges from 54% to 91%. When chemoradiation is used as the primary modality, the 2-year survival ranges from 52% to 81%.

## Summary

There is a plethora of management techniques for advanced laryngeal cancer. The decision to proceed with surgical or nonsurgical management needs to be made according to the patient's wishes and quality-of-life goals and with input from the medical oncologists, radiation oncologists, and head and neck surgeons. The much-discussed total laryngectomy of the past is now relegated to T4 cases with extensions into neighboring areas and for salvage in recurrent cases. For cases with distant metastases (M1) palliation is the only treatment the physician can offer. Partial laryngectomy techniques are gaining popularity again, but large, randomized trials to compare the voice quality and oncologic control still need to be performed. Chemoradiation therapy protocols have allowed nonsurgical management, but their judicious use is advocated because surgical salvage for failures is both complicated and morbid. Organ preservation does not equate with preservation of organ function. Therefore surgery should not be abandoned or considered as the last option in patients with advanced laryngeal cancer but should remain as a primary therapy in these patients.

## References


[1] Larynx. In: The American Joint Committee on Cancer cancer staging manual. 5th edition. Philadelphia: Lippincott-Raven; 1997. p. 41–6.

[2] Birmingham & West Midland Cancer Registry, 1986. In: Kerr A, Grove J, editors. Scott-Brown's otolaryngology. 5th edition. London: Butterworths; 1987. p. 195.

[3] Powel J, Robin PE. Cancer of head and neck: the present state. In: Rhys E, Robin PE, Fielding JWL, editors. Head & neck cancer. Turnbridge Wells (UK): Castle House Publications; 1983. p. 3–16.

[4] Broders AC. Practical points on the microscopic grading of carcinoma. N Y State J Med 1932;32:667–71.

[5] Ogura JH. Surgical pathology of carcinoma of larynx. Laryngoscope 1955;65:867–926.

[6] Ampil FL, Nathan CA, Caldito G, et al. Total laryngectomy and postoperative radiotherapy for T4 laryngeal cancer: a 14 year review. Am J Otolaryngol 2004;25:88–93.

[7] Lefebvre JL, Lartigau E. Preservation of form and function during management of cancer of the larynx and hypo-pharynx. World J Surg 2003;27:811–6.

[8] Jalisi M. Our first three laryngectomies. J Laryngol Otol 1965;79:824–7.

[9] Weinstein GS. Surgical approach to organ preservation in the treatment of carcinoma of larynx. Oncology 2001;15:785–96.

[10] Lederman M. Radiotherapy of the cancer of the larynx. J Laryngol Otol 1970;84(9):867–96.

[11] Ferlito A, Silver CE, Howard DJ, et al. The role of partial laryngeal resection in current management of laryngeal cancer: a collective review. Acta Otolaryngol 2000;120(4):456–65.

[12] Davis RK, Kriskovich MD, Galloway EB III, et al. Endoscopic supraglottic laryngectomy with postoperative irradiation. Ann Otol Rhinol Laryngol 2004;113(2):132–8.

[13] Harrison DF. The pathology and management of subglottic cancer. Ann Otol Rhinol Laryngol 1971;80(1):6–12.

[14] Bryce DP. The role of surgery in the management of carcinoma of the larynx. J Laryngol Otol 1972;86:669–83.

[15] Price LA, Hill BT. Chemotherapy in head and neck cancer. In: Scott-Brown's otolaryngology. 5th edition. London: Butterworths; 1987. p. 498–512.

[16] Radcliffe G, Shaw HJ. Partial laryngectomy for recurrent cancer after irradiation. Clinical Otolaryngology 1978;3:49–62.

[17] Stell PM, Dalby JE, Singh SD, et al. The management of glottic T3 carcinoma. Clin Otolaryngol 1982;7(3):175–80.

[18] Hill BT, Price LA. The potential role of chemotherapy in improving survival in some common cancers. Pharmacy International 1984;5:268–72.

[19] Kisch JA, Ensley JF, Weaver A, et al. Improvement of complete response rate to induction adjuvant chemotherapy for advanced squamous cell carcinoma of the head and neck. In: Jones SE, Salmon SE, editors. Adjuvant therapy of cancer IV. New York: Grune & Stratton; 1985. p. 107–115.
[20] Jacob C, Wolf G, Mahuch R. Adjuvant chemotherapy for head and neck squamous carcinomas. Proceedings of the American Society of Clinical Oncology 1984;3:182.
[21] Sewell DA. Supracricoid partial laryngectomy with cricohyoidopexy. Operative Techniques in Otolaryngology Head and Neck Surgery 2003;14:27–33.
[22] Rassekh CH, Johnson JT. Controversies in management of the N0 neck in squamous cell carcinoma of the upper aerodigestive tract. In: Bailey BJ, Calhoun KH, Healy GB, et al, editors. Head and neck surgery-otolaryngology. 3rd edition. Philadelphia: Lippincott Williams and Wilkins; 2001. p. 1367–75.
[23] American Head and Neck Society. Tumors of the upper aerodigestive tract: larynx-supraglottic. Available at: www.headandneckcancer.org/clinical/resources/docs/supralarynx.php. Accessed November 4, 2004.
[24] Ferlito A, Shaha AR, Lefebvre JL, et al. Organ and voice preservation in advanced laryngeal cancer. Acta Otolaryngol 2002;122:438–42.
[25] Garden AS. Organ preservation for carcinoma of the larynx and hypopharynx. Hematol Oncol Clin North Am 2001;15:243–60.
[26] The Department of Veterans Affairs Laryngeal Cancer Study Group. Induction chemotherapy plus radiation compared with surgery plus radiation in patients with advanced laryngeal cancer. N Engl J Med 1991;324:1685–90.
[27] DeSanto LW. Cancer of the larynx. Curr Opin Otolaryngol Head Neck Surg 1993;1:133–6.
[28] Moyer JS, Wolf GT, Bradford CR. Current thoughts on the role of chemotherapy and radiation in advanced head and neck cancer. Curr Opin Otol Head Neck Surg 2004;12:82–7.
[29] Hillman RE, Walsh M, Wolf GT, et al. Functional outcomes following treatment for advanced laryngeal cancer: part 1: voice preservation in advanced laryngeal cancer. Ann Otol Rhinol Laryngol 1998;172:1–27.
[30] Terrell JE, Fisher SG, Wolf GT, et al. Long term quality of life after treatment for laryngeal cancer. Arch Otolaryngol Head Neck Surg 1998;124:964–71.
[31] Forastiere AA, Berkey B, Maor M, et al. Phase III trial to preserve the larynx: induction chemotherapy and radiotherapy versus concomitant chemoradiotherapy versus radiotherapy alone, Intergroup Trial R91-11 [abstract]. Proc Am Soc Clin Oncol 2001:20: abstract 4.
[32] Keum KC, Kim GE, Suh CO, et al. Role of definitive radiation therapy for larynx preservation in patients with advanced laryngeal cancer. J Otolarngol 1999;28:245–51.
[33] Kraus DH, Pfister DG, Harrison LB, et al. Salvage laryngectomy for unsuccessful larynx preservation therapy. Ann Otol Rhinol Laryngol 1995;104:936–41.
[34] Sassler AM, Esclamado RM, Wolf GT. Surgery after organ preservation therapy: analysis of wound complications. Arch Otolaryngol Head Neck Surg 1995;121:162–5.

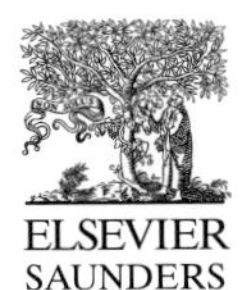

ELSEVIER
SAUNDERS

Otolaryngol Clin N Am
38 (2005) 59–74

OTOLARYNGOLOGIC
CLINICS
OF NORTH AMERICA


# Squamous Cell Carcinoma of the Oropharynx and Hypopharynx


Derrick T. Lin, MD[a], Seth M. Cohen, MD, MPH[b],*,
George L. Coppit, MD[c], Brian B. Burkey, MD[b]

[a]*Department of Otolaryngology, Massachusetts Eye and Ear Infirmary,
243 Charles Street, Boston, MA 02114, USA*
[b]*Department of Otolaryngology, Vanderbilt University Medical Center,
1301 22nd Avenue South, Nashville, TN 37212, USA*
[c]*Department of Otolaryngology, Walter Reed Army Medical Centers,
6th Floor 6B 7100 Georgia Avenue, Washington DC, 20307, USA*


## Oropharyngeal cancer

### Surgical anatomy

The oropharynx incorporates an area that extends from the junction of the soft palate and hard palate superiorly to the circumvallate papillae of the tongue anteriorly and to the hyoid bone inferiorly. The subsites of the oropharynx include the soft palate, base of tongue, tonsillar fossa and pillars, and a portion of the posterior pharyngeal wall. There are approximately 5000 newly diagnosed oropharyngeal cancers per year in the United States with squamous cell carcinoma being by far the most common histologic type [1]. The most important causative factors are prolonged tobacco and alcohol exposure.

There are potential fascial spaces that surround the oropharynx. Lying deep to the mucosal layer are the thick intrinsic muscles of the tongue base and the thin muscular layers of the superior and middle pharyngeal constrictors, which act as partial barriers to tumor spread. When invasion does occur, tumors may spread into the potential spaces of the neck. The retropharyngeal space lies posterior to these structures and represents a potential site for tumor extension, as does the more posteriorly placed prevertebral muscles and fascia. A second potential space for tumor extension is the parapharyngeal space lateral to the pharyngeal constrictors that forms

---


* Corresponding author.
*E-mail address:* seth.cohen@vanderbilt.edu (S.M. Cohen).

an inverted pyramid with its base at the skull and its apex at the greater cornu of the hyoid bone. The parapharyngeal space contains branches of the trigeminal nerve, pterygoid muscles, and the internal maxillary artery.

Functionally, the oropharynx is critical for proper speech production, respiration, and deglutition. During swallowing, the soft palate acts by closing the nasopharynx from the oropharynx, thus preventing nasopharyngeal regurgitation. This function is also critical for preventing hypernasal speech. The base of tongue acts in concert by propelling the food bolus into the hypopharynx. Because of these important functions, surgical resection of oropharyngeal cancers may result in poor speech production, dysphagia, or aspiration. Proper patient selection for surgical therapy, appropriate reconstruction, and postoperative care are therefore critical for optimal care of patients with oropharyngeal cancer.

*Presentation*

Cancers of the oropharynx occur most frequently in patients older than 45 years of age and have a strong association with tobacco smoke and alcohol use [2–5]. When present, the most common symptom is throat discomfort. Symptoms occur earlier in lesions of the soft palate than in cancers of the tonsil or base of tongue. Other complaints include odynophagia, a globus sensation, and otalgia. With invasion of deep musculature, trismus, dysphagia, and dysarthria may develop. Additional late symptoms include bleeding, aspiration, airway obstruction, and weight loss.

Oropharyngeal cancers tend to be asymptomatic in the early stages. In fact, patients with oropharyngeal cancer may initially present with a neck mass. Depending on the subsite, 45% to 78% of patients with oropharyngeal primaries may present with cervical adenopathy at the time of diagnosis [6].

*Base of tongue*

Persistent sore throat is the most common presenting symptom of base of tongue cancers, representing 40% to 80% of cases. The base of tongue, however, is often difficult to visualize, and submucosal lesions are common. Digital palpation of the tongue base in patients with persistent sore throat is thus critical in making a proper diagnosis. Squamous cell carcinoma of the base of tongue commonly presents at an advanced stage with high rates of cervical and distant metastasis. The overall survival rate has been reported to be as low as 20% [7–9]. Squamous cell carcinomas of the base of tongue are clinically distinct from cancers of the oral tongue, in general being more aggressive. Furthermore, most cancers of the tongue base are of a relatively high grade, with 60% to 90% being poorly or moderately differentiated. If disease is detected early, survival rates of 50% to 60% can still be achieved [7–9].

The incidence of cervical lymph node metastasis in squamous cell carcinoma of the tongue base is high, even in T1 and T2 lesions [7,8]. Lymph node metastases most commonly involve levels II, III, and IV of the neck. More than 60% of patients with cancer of the base of tongue have at least one clinically involved node at the time of presentation. Almost 20% present with bilateral cervical metastases secondary to the rich lymphatic system of the base of tongue. As in other sites, the presence of cervical metastases decreases survival by more than 50% [8,9]. Although distant metastases are rare at the time of presentation, if locoregional disease is not controlled, distant metastases eventually become evident in 30% to 50% of patients [8–11].

*Soft palate*

Approximately 15% of cancers of the soft palate are found during routine physical examination. When present, the most common chief complaint is odynophagia. Cancers in this location are most commonly present on the anterior surface of the soft palate. They tend to be visible and symptomatic earlier than other cancers of the oropharynx. Russ et al [12] reported in their series that 21% of patients presented at stage I (T1 N0), 34% presented at stage II (T2 N0), 25% presented at stage III, and only 13% presented at stage IV.

The rate of clinically positive cervical lymph node metastases ranges from 2% to 45% at the time of presentation. These metastases are bilateral in 5% to 15% of patients with primary lymphatic drainage to level II [13].

*Tonsil*

The tonsillar fossa and tonsillar pillars are the most common sites of squamous cell carcinoma of the oropharynx, contributing 75% to 80% of all squamous cell carcinomas of the oropharynx. They tend to be asymptomatic early in their clinical course, but 60% to 80% of patients present with odynophagia or dysphagia, whereas 10% to 38% present with only suspicious adenopathy [14]. Other symptoms include otalgia, globus sensation, or bleeding. Posterior and deep extension may involve the pterygoid musculature causing significant pain and trismus [15–17].

Squamous cell carcinoma of the tonsil most often presents with involvement of the anterior tonsillar pillar. These cancers are often exophytic and frequently spread anteriorly or medially to involve the retromolar trigone, buccal, and tongue base mucosa. In fact, tongue base extension has been reported in 41% to 80% of patients. In contrast, extension posteriorly onto the pharyngeal wall occurs much less commonly [16,18].

Because these lesions infiltrate deeply, the lingual nerve, inferior alveolar nerve, glossopharyngeal nerve, and mandible may become involved just deep to the anterior tonsillar pillar. Eventual involvement of the pterygoid musculature and parapharyngeal space will cause significant trismus.

Clinically positive lymph node metastasis at presentation has been reported to be between 66% and 76% [15,18,19]. This metastasis most often occurs in regions II, III, and IV. Metastases to contralateral lymph nodes occur in up to 22% of tonsillar fossa lesions and in 6% of lesions of the anterior tonsillar pillar [20,21].

### Posterior and lateral oropharyngeal walls

Squamous cell carcinoma of the pharyngeal wall frequently presents at an advanced stage. Cunningham et al [22] reported that 78% of these cancers presented at a size greater than 5 cm. They often extend either superiorly to the nasopharynx or inferiorly to the hypopharynx. The most common symptoms of cancer of the posterior pharyngeal wall are dysphagia (66%) and odynophagia (62%). Other symptoms include weight loss, neck pain, and hoarseness. Initial presentation of a neck mass was reported in 20% of patients.

### Evaluation and staging

The first step in evaluating a patient with possible oropharyngeal cancer includes a thorough history and physical examination. The size and mobility of the lesion should be documented. The presence of trismus or decreased mobility of the tongue is a sign of invasion of the pterygomaxillary space or deep tongue muscles. A thorough examination of cranial nerves should be performed, specifically of cranial nerves V, VII, XI, X, and XII. The number and size of lymph nodes should be evaluated.

CT or MRI may be useful in select patients. MRI is useful for evaluating soft tissue involvement, particularly of the tongue base and the para-pharyngeal space and especially in patients who are difficult to examine. CT, on the other hand, is useful in evaluating invasion of bone of the skull base or mandible. Patients should have a chest radiograph and liver function tests for metastatic screening. The role of positron emission tomographic scanning is currently being evaluated, but this modality is probably not beneficial routinely.

Patients with suspected oropharyngeal carcinoma should be evaluated under general anesthesia for tumor staging, tissue biopsy, and to screen for second primary tumors. The current American Joint Committee on Cancer (AJCC) staging system is shown in Box 1.

### Treatment

Surgery, radiation therapy, and chemoradiation therapy, individually or in combination, are the mainstays of treatment for squamous cell carcinoma of the oropharynx. An interdisciplinary approach that includes head and neck surgeons, radiation oncologists, medical oncologists, and speech and swallow pathologists are essential in the optimal treatment of patients with oropharyngeal carcinoma. Several factors must be considered in the treatment of oropharyngeal carcinomas including stage of disease, aggressiveness of the histology of the tumor, comorbid medical conditions, and patients' and families' wishes.

**Box 1. American Joint Committee on Cancer staging for oropharyngeal carcinoma [23]**

*Tumor*
T1 Tumor 2 cm or less in greatest dimension
T2 Tumor more than 2 cm but not more than 4 cm in greatest dimension
T3 Tumor more than 4 cm in greatest dimension
T4a Tumor invades the larynx, deep/extrinsic muscle of tongue, medial pterygoid, hard palate, or mandible
T4b Tumor invades lateral pterygoid muscle, pterygoid plates, lateral nasopharynx, or skull base or encases carotid artery

*Regional lymph nodes*
NX Regional lymph nodes cannot be assessed
N0 No regional lymph node metastasis
N1 Metastasis in a single ipsilateral lymph node 3 cm or less in greatest dimension
N2 Metastasis in a single ipsilateral lymph node more than 3 cm but not more than 6 cm in greatest dimension, or in multiple ipsilateral lymph nodes, none more than 6 cm in greatest dimension, or in bilateral or contralateral lymph nodes, none more than 6 cm in greatest dimension
N2a Metastasis in a single ipsilateral lymph node more than 3 cm but not more than 6 cm in greatest dimension
N2b Metastasis in multiple ipsilateral lymph nodes, none more than 6 cm in greatest dimension
N2c Metastasis in bilateral or contralateral lymph nodes, none more than 6 cm in greatest dimension
N3 Metastasis in a lymph node more than 6 cm in greatest dimension

*Distant metastasis*
MX Distant metastasis cannot be assessed
M0 No distant metastasis
M1 Distant metastasis

*Stage grouping*
Stage 0 Tis N0 M0
Stage I T1 N0 M0
Stage II T2 N0 M0
Stage III T3 N0 M0
T1 N1 M0
T2 N1 M0
T3 N1 M0

Stage IVA T4a N0 M0
T4a N1 M0
T1 N2 M0
T2 N2 M0
T3 N2 M0
T4a N2 M0
Stage IVB T4b Any N M0
Any T N3 M0
Stage IVC Any T Any N M1

---

*Adapted from* the American Joint Committee on Cancer cancer staging manual. 6th edition. New York: Springer-Verlag; 2002.

An argument can be made against primary surgical therapy for oropharyngeal cancers. Even early-stage carcinomas are at risk for regional lymph node metastases. Traditional neck dissections often fail to address retropharyngeal and parapharyngeal lymphatics, which are at risk in patients with oropharyngeal carcinoma. In addition, there is a high risk of bilateral neck disease in these patients. Because of these issues and the morbidity of surgical resection of the oropharynx, there has been an overall trend toward primary therapy with radiation or chemoradiation therapy, especially for advanced disease.

Single-modality therapy with radiation or surgery can achieve similar locoregional control for early and intermediate cancers, with radiotherapy generally yielding better functional outcomes [24]. A large percentage of patients undergoing primary surgical resection require postoperative radiation therapy because of the presence of positive nodes, extracapsular spread, or perineural invasion. Several studies have reported improved locoregional and overall disease-free survival in patients receiving postoperative radiation therapy versus surgical treatment alone [25–28]. Many institutions therefore recommend radiation therapy for early-stage disease and chemoradiation therapy for intermediate- and advanced-stage disease.

*Surgical approaches*

In general, surgical treatment of oropharyngeal carcinomas is typically reserved for patients who have failed primary radiation or chemoradiation therapy and for those who for any reason are not candidates for such therapy. The key factor in any approach is adequate exposure. Generally, all approaches are accompanied by a neck dissection.

Transoral approaches to the oropharynx are the simplest, but success depends on the size and location of the tumor. When possible, a transoral approach is the preferred method for excising smaller lesions of the soft palate, posterior pharyngeal wall, tonsil and anterior pillar, and uvula. Recently, transoral laser approaches have been described for treatment of small lesions of the base of tongue [29].

The mandibular swing approach provides wide exposure of the entire oropharynx when the transoral approach is inadequate and the mandible is not involved. Mandibular osteotomies are performed anterior to the mental foramen, preserving the sensory innervation of the lip and chin [30]. The floor of mouth is released along with the lateralized mandibular segment, while preserving the lingual nerve in its course if uninvolved, and so creating wide exposure to the oropharynx. For oropharyngeal cancers that involve the mandible, composite resection of the mandible and oropharynx may be required. This resection is achieved with by lip-splitting or a visor flap incision [31].

The transcervical transpharyngeal approaches include a suprahyoid approach and a lateral pharyngotomy approach. These approaches have the advantage of minimally disrupting existing functional anatomy while providing adequate exposure for selected posterior oropharyngeal tumors. They may be combined, if necessary, for exposure but require some experience to be used effectively. The suprahyoid approach is most appropriate for small neoplasms of the midline base of tongue. A cervical incision is required, followed by entering the pharynx above the hyoid bone into the vallecula [32]. The tumor is excised inferiorly to superiorly. The lateral pharyngotomy approach differs in that the pharynx is entered between the hypoglossal and superior laryngeal nerves. A rather limited view of the tongue base can be improved by extending into a suprahyoid approach, thus giving an excellent view of the base of tongue and pharyngeal walls. This approach is usually inadequate for lesions extending superiorly to the tonsillar fossa or retromolar trigone region.

*Reconstruction of the oropharynx*

Options for reconstruction range from primary closure to microvascular free flap tissue transfer. The objective of reconstruction is to restore functional speech and swallowing while providing an adequate airway. The simplest method of reconstruction, primary closure, is reserved for small defects where minimal tethering will be created, such as early lesions of the base of tongue where transpharyngeal approaches have been employed. The next option in the reconstructive ladder is the use of skin grafting. This technique is usually limited to lesions along the posterior and lateral pharyngeal wall where a bolster can be placed.

The most commonly used pedicled regional flap is the pectoralis major myocutaneous flap. It is extremely reliable and provides sufficient bulk to fill major defects of the oropharynx [32,33]. Other pedicled flaps described for reconstruction of the oropharynx include the latissimus dorsi flap and the trapezius myocutaneous flap [34,35]. In general, primary closure and split-thickness skin graft are reserved for smaller lesions, whereas flaps are used for larger defects. Pedicled flaps work best where mobility and sensation are less critical, such as in the tonsil and lateral pharyngeal regions.

Microvascular free tissue transfer represents the highest level of sophistication for reconstruction of the oropharynx. The radial forearm flap, based on the radial artery, provides a thin, pliable, and possibly sensate reconstructive option [36]. The lateral arm flap, based on the posterior radial collateral artery, is another option for reconstruction of the oropharynx. This flap is unique in that the lower half of the flap is thin, but the upper half has additional bulk, making it ideal for tongue base reconstruction in conjunction with adjacent palate or pharynx [37]. These flaps are most effectively used in tongue base and palatal defects where mobility is essential to function. When the mandible is invaded and a mandibulectomy is required, bony microvascular free tissue may be used such as the fibular or scapular osteofasciocutaneous free flap.

## Chemoradiation therapy

Single-modality therapy with radiation or surgery can achieve similar locoregional control rates for early-stage cancers. With advanced disease, there has been a trend toward combination chemoradiation therapy. Traditionally, patients with stage III and IV disease have been treated with surgery followed by radiation therapy with disappointing survival rates ranging from 30% to 40% [37,38]. Concomitant or induction chemotherapy is in theory an attractive option for treatment of oropharyngeal cancer. The addition of chemotherapy may provide better regional and distant tumor control. Concurrent chemotherapy markedly enhances the cytotoxicity of radiation therapy. Several prospective, randomized studies have addressed the efficacy of concomitant chemoradiation therapy versus radiation therapy alone for advanced-stage squamous cell carcinoma of the head and neck (Table 1). In general, these studies provide strong data demonstrating a statistically significant improvement in locoregional control and a strong trend for improved overall survival with concomitant chemoradiation therapy over radiation therapy alone for patients with advanced oropharyngeal carcinoma.

## Hypopharyngeal carcinoma

### Surgical anatomy

The hypopharynx is a region continuous with the oropharynx extending from the level of the hyoid bone to the esophageal inlet. It is intimately associated with the larynx, surrounding its posterior and lateral borders. The subsites of the hypopharynx include the pyriform sinus, the posterior

Table 1
Studies of concomitant chemoradiation

| Study | Patients | Experimental arms | Conclusions |
| --- | --- | --- | --- |
| Denis [65] (n = 226) | Stage III/IV oropharynx | Standard fractionation RT vs concomitant RT + carboplatin + 5 fluorouracil | Concommitant chemoradiation therapy showed improved overall survival and locoregional control rates and does not statistically increase late morbidity. |
| Wendt [66] (n = 270) | Stage III/IV (oropharynx, oral cavity, larynx, hypopharynx) | Accelerated fractionation RT vs concomitant RT + cisplatin + 5 fluorouracil + leukovorin | Concommitant chemoradiation therapy showed improved disease control and survival however with increased acute toxicity. |
| Brizel [67] (n = 116) relapse | Unresectable HNSCC | Hyperfractionated RT vs concomitant RT + cisplatin + 5 fluorouracil | Concurrent chemoradiation therapy showed improved overall survival, disease-free survival, and locoregional control. Nearly half of these patients ultimately died of disease. |
| Jeremic [68] (n = 159) | Stage III/IV HNSCC | Standard fractionation RT vs concomitant RT + cisplatin (CDPP) vs concomitant RT + carboplatin (CBDCA) | CDPP and CBDCA groups had improved median survival time, median time to local recurrence, 5-year local recurrence-free survival, and 5-year overall survival. There was no difference between CDPP and CBDCA groups. |

*Abbreviations:* HNSCC, head and neck squamous cell carcinoma; RT, radiation therapy.

pharyngeal wall, and the postcricoid region. The superior aspect of the pyriform sinus is surrounded by the thyrohyoid membrane through which the internal branch of the superior laryngeal nerve passes. Sensory portions of this nerve synapse along with sensory nerves of the external auditory canal (Arnold's nerve) leading to symptoms of referred otalgia. The postcricoid region lies posterior to the arytenoid cartilages and cricoid ring, terminating at the junction between the pharynx and esophagus. The posterior pharyngeal wall of the hypopharynx begins at the level of the hyoid bone continuing also to the pharyngoesophageal junction.

Cancers of the hypopharynx are uncommon, representing only about 0.5% of all malignancies. As with cancers of the oropharynx, most cancers of the hypopharynx are squamous cell carcinoma in histology and have a strong association with alcohol and tobacco abuse and, more recently, with chronic reflux disease [39]. Of note, patients with Plummer-Vinson syndrome are at high risk of developing cancers in the postcricoid region [40].

Cancers arising from the medial wall of the pyriform sinus may extend toward the aryepiglottic fold or arytenoids. They may invade deeply into the cricoarytenoid joint, paraglottic, and pre-epiglottic space leading to vocal cord fixation. Lesions of the lateral pyriform wall tend to spread to the posterior pharynx but may spread more deeply to involve the thyroid ala or may continue inferiorly to the ipsilateral thyroid gland. Tumors arising in the postcricoid region commonly invade into the posterior cricoarytenoid muscles and cricoid, whereas lesions of the posterior pharyngeal wall may spread superiorly to the nasopharynx, inferiorly to the cervical esophagus, or deeply to the prevertebral muscles and retropharyngeal space.

The hypopharynx has a rich lymphatic supply with its major lymphatic drainage pattern to the jugular chain [41]. There is also significant lymphatic drainage to the retropharyngeal lymph nodes and the node of Rouviere [42].

*Clinical presentation*

The most common presenting symptoms of patients with hypopharyngeal carcinoma are sore throat, dysphagia, otalgia, hoarseness, or a neck mass. Patients also frequently complain of a globus sensation and weight loss. Approximately 25% of patients with hypopharyngeal cancer present with symptoms of a neck mass, whereas 70% of patients will have palpable adenopathy on initial examination [43,44].

*Evaluation and staging*

A thorough history and physical examination are critical in the evaluation of patients with suspected hypopharyngeal squamous cell carcinoma. Indirect pharyngolaryngoscopy with the laryngeal mirror remains vital to proper evaluation. Tumors of the posterior wall or upper pyriform sinus are usually readily visualized by this method. When necessary, flexible fiberoptic examination may be used. Lesions in the apex of the pyriform sinus and postcricoid region may often be obscured and difficult to visualize in the office setting. Edema, erythema, pooling of secretions, and loss of laryngeal crepitus are important signs of hypopharyngeal carcinoma. Vocal cord mobility should be assessed because laryngeal invasion with limited vocal cord mobility is a sign of more extensive disease. Palpation of the neck is necessary for evaluation of lymphadenopathy.

Patients with suspected hypopharyngeal cancer should undergo direct laryngoscopy, esophagoscopy, and biopsy under general anesthesia to facilitate accurate evaluation and staging as well as allowing identification of possible synchronous tumors. The AJCC classification system for hypopharyngeal carcinoma is shown in Box 2.

CT and MRI scans are important imaging modalities in the initial evaluation of patients with hypopharyngeal carcinoma. These studies allow

**Box 2. American Joint Committee on Cancer staging for hypopharyngeal carcinoma [23]**

T1 Tumor limited to one subsite of hypopharynx and 2 cm or less in greatest dimension

T2 Tumor invades more than one subsite of hypopharynx or an adjacent site, or measures more than 2 cm but not more than 4 cm in greatest diameter without fixation of hemilarynx

T3 Tumor more than 4 cm in greatest dimension or with fixation of hemilarynx

T4a Tumor invades thyroid/cricoid cartilage, hyoid bone, thyroid gland, esophagus, or central compartment soft tissue

T4b Tumor invades prevertebral fascia, encases carotid artery, or involves mediastinal structures

N staging, M staging and stage grouping is same as for oropharynx

---

*Adapted from* the American Joint Committee on Cancer cancer staging manual. 6th edition. New York: Springer-Verlag; 2002.

further evaluation of the primary site (eg, for laryngeal cartilage erosion) as well as evaluation for the presence of cervical lymphadenopathy.

## Treatment

### Surgery

Appropriate therapy for tumors of the hypopharynx is predicated on several factors. The patient's performance status, extent of disease, laryngeal involvement, and the presence of lymph node metastasis must be taken into account. Only very select patients with tumors of the hypopharynx are amenable to conservation laryngeal surgery. Early lesions of the pharyngeal wall may be treated with surgical resection, but preservation of the larynx has been reported to be possible in less than 50% of cases [45]. Small T1 and T2 tumors arising from the medial wall of the pyriform sinus may be amenable to a laryngeal preservation procedure. Contraindications include thyroid cartilage invasion, involvement of the apex of the pyriform sinus, involvement of the postcricoid region, and impairment of vocal cord motion. For lesions of the postcricoid region, laryngectomy is almost always required. Despite an increasing trend toward organ preservation, total laryngectomy with partial or total pharyngectomy followed by postoperative radiation therapy are the most common surgical procedures performed for advanced squamous cell carcinoma of the hypopharynx [46–48].

If primary surgical therapy is recommended, elective neck dissection should be performed at the time of surgery because of the high incidence of bilateral occult cervical metastasis [49–51]. In addition, retropharyngeal nodes are involved in almost 50% of patients with pharyngeal cancers and should also be addressed at the time of surgery [52].

*Surgical reconstruction*

Primary closure or skin grafting may be used for small defects. Posterior pharyngeal wall lesions have been described as being the most amenable to skin grafting [53]. The pectoralis major myocutaneous flap or radial forearm free flap may be used for reconstruction of subtotal hypopharyngeal defects in which a posterior strip of mucosa is left after the ablative procedure [54,55]. For lesions of the hypopharynx that require total laryngophar- yngectomy, a free jejunal flap or a tubed radial forearm free flap provides an excellent method of reconstruction [56]. In a total laryngopharyngectomy defect where the distal esophageal stump lies inferior to the sternal notch, gastric interposition may be required. This procedure, however, requires major abdominal surgery and extensive mediastinal dissection. Operative morbidity is nearly 50%, and mortality rates have been reported to reach 10% [57].

*Chemotherapy and radiation therapy*

Radiation therapy has been proposed for treatment of hypopharyngeal cancers. For early-stage disease, results comparable to conservation surgical treatment have been reported [58]. On the other hand, with advanced disease, control rates with radiation therapy alone were inferior to surgery combined with postoperative radiation therapy [59–61].

An organ-preservation protocol using chemotherapy is another option for improving results of therapy for advanced disease. The European Organization for Research and Treatment of Cancer [62] conducted a randomized trial evaluating treatment of advanced squamous cell carcinoma of the hypopharynx. This study compared surgery and post- operative radiation therapy with induction chemotherapy followed by radiation. If there was no response to the induction chemotherapy in the experimental arm, surgery was performed and was followed by post- operative radiation therapy, but a complete response after induction chemotherapy was followed by definitive radiation therapy. This study found a survival advantage in the experimental arm at 3-year follow-up but not at 5 years, with 50% of the survivors in the experimental arm having preserved the larynx at both time points.

In 1997 Beauvillain et al [63] published their data comparing patients with resectable cancer of the hypopharynx who were amenable only to total laryngopharyngectomy with patients randomly assigned to receive in- duction chemotherapy. Specifically, one arm consisted of chemotherapy followed by surgery and radiation therapy, and the second arm consisted of chemotherapy followed by radiation therapy, reserving surgery for salvage. They concluded that patients in the surgical arm had better local control

(63%) and 5-year survival (37%) than patients in the nonsurgical arm (19% 5-year survival and 39% local control), suggesting that tumor response to chemotherapy may need to be taken into account before radiation therapy is chosen instead of surgery.

Given all the data, the mainstay of treatment in advanced cancer of the hypopharynx remains surgery followed by radiation therapy, with chemo-radiation therapy regimens used in selected situations and in controlled trials. The overall prognosis for patients with squamous cell carcinoma of the hypopharynx is poor because most of these patients present at an advanced stage, and many patients succumb to distant disease. Overall, patients with late-stage hypopharyngeal carcinoma treated with curative intent have a 5-year survival of approximately 35% [64].

## Summary

Treating oropharyngeal and hypopharyngeal squamous cell carcinomas presents challenges for the head and neck oncologist. A thorough evaluation is necessary to stage these tumors appropriately. Surgical treatment requires addressing the primary tumor and also neck disease, reconstructive techniques, and associated morbidities. Alternatively, chemoradiation organ-preservation protocols have been increasingly used in the treatment of advanced head and neck cancer. A multidisciplinary approach helps balance the tumor stage, patient comorbidities, functional outcome, and patient wishes, thereby maximizing patient outcomes.

## References

[1] Greenlee RT, Hill-Harmon MB, Murray T, et al. Cancer statistics, 2001. Ca J Clin 2001;51: 15–36.
[2] Blot WJ, McLaughlin JD, Winn DM, et al. Smoking and drinking in relation to oral and pharyngeal cancer. Cancer Res 1988;37:4608.
[3] Wynder EL, Stellman SD. Comparative epidemiology of tobacco-related cancers. Cancer Res 1977;37:4608.
[4] Schottendfield D, Gantt RD, Wynder EL. The role of alcohol and tobacco in multiple primary cancers of the upper digestive system, larynx, and lung: a prospective study. Prev Med 1974;3:277.
[5] Moore C. Cigarette smoking and cancer of the mouth, pharynx, and larynx. JAMA 1971; 218:553.
[6] Lindberg R. Distribution of cervical lymph node metastasis from squamous cell carcinoma of the upper respiratory and digestive tracts. Cancer 1972;29:1446–9.
[7] Weber PC, Myers EN, Johnson JT. Squamous cell carcinoma of the base of the tongue. Eur Arch Otorhinolaryngol 1993;250:63–8.
[8] Callery CD, Spiro R, Strong EH. Changing trends in the management of squamous cell carcinoma of the tongue base. Am J Surg 1984;148:449–54.
[9] Schleunig AJ, Summers GW. Carcinoma of the tongue: review of 220 cases. Laryngoscope 1972;82:1446–54.

[10] Close LG, Merkel M, Vuitch MF, et al. Computed tomographic evaluation of regional lymph node involvement in cancer of the oral cavity and oropharynx. Head Neck 1989;11:309–17.

[11] Foote RL, Olsen KD, Davis DL, et al. Base of tongue carcinoma: patterns of failure and predictors of recurrence after surgery alone. Head Neck 1993;15:300–7.

[12] Russ JE, Applebaum EL, Sisson GA. Squamous cell carcinoma of the palate. Laryngoscope 1977;87:1151–6.

[13] Hussey DH, Latourette HB, Panje WR. Head and neck cancer: an analysis of the incidence, patterns of treatment, and survival at the University of Iowa. Ann Otol Rhinol Laryngol Suppl 1991;152:2–16.

[14] Cancer statistics 1993. CA Cancer J Clin 1993;43:18.

[15] Martin H, Sugarbaker E. Cancer of the tonsil. Am J Surg 1941;52:158–97.

[16] Perez CA, Mill WB, Ogura JH, et al. Carcinoma of the tonsil: sequential comparisons of four treatment modalities. Radiology 1970;94:649–59.

[17] Fleming PM, Matz GJ, Powell WI, et al. Carcinoma of the tonsil. Surg Clin North Am 1976;56:125–36.

[18] Petrovich Z, Kuisk H, Jose L, et al. Advanced carcinoma of the tonsil: treatment results. Acta Radiol Oncol 1980;19:425–31.

[19] Zelefsky MJ, Harrison LB, Armstrong JG. Long-term treatment results of postoperative radiation therapy for advanced oropharyngeal carcinoma. Cancer 1993;70:2388–95.

[20] Micheau C, Cachin Y, Caillou B. Cystic metastases in the neck revealing occult carcinoma of the tonsil: a report of 6 cases. Cancer 1974;33:228–33.

[21] Jesse RH Jr, Fletcher GH. Metastases in cervical lymph nodes from oropharyngeal carcinoma: treatment and results. AJR Am J Roentgenol 1963;90:990–6.

[22] Cunningham MP, Catlin D. Cancer of the pharyngeal wall. Cancer 1967;20:1859–66.

[23] Greene FL, Page DL, Fleming ID, et al. AJCC cancer staging manual. 6th edition. New York: Springer-Verlag; 2002.

[24] Weber RS, Peters LG, Wolf P, et al. Squamous cell carcinoma of the soft palate, uvula, and anterior faucial pillar. Otolaryngol Head Neck Surg 1988;99:16–23.

[25] Weber RS, Gidley P, Morrison WH, et al. Treatment selection for carcinoma of the base of the tongue. Am J Surg 1990;160:415–9.

[26] Kraus DH, Vastola AP, Huvos AG, et al. Surgical management of squamous cell carcinoma of the base of the tongue. Am J Surg 1993;166:384–8.

[27] Zelefsky MJ, Harrison LB, Armstrong JG. Long-term treatment results of postoperative radiation therapy for advanced stage oropharyngeal carcinoma. Cancer 1993;70:2388–95.

[28] Perez CA, Carmichael T, Devenini VR, et al. Carcinoma of the tonsillar fossa: a non-randomized comparison of irradiation alone or combined with surgery: long term results. Head Neck 1991;13:282–90.

[29] Steiner W, Ambrosch P, Hess CF, et al. Organ preservation by transoral laser microsurgery in pyriform sinus carcinoma. Otolaryngol Head Neck Surg 2001;124:58–67.

[30] Clayman GL, Adams GL. Modifications of the mandibular swing for preservation of occlusion and function. Head Neck 1991;13:102–6.

[31] La Ferriere JA, Sessions DG, Thawley SE, et al. A functional approach to composite resection and reconstruction for cancer of the oral cavity and oropharynx. Arch Otolaryngol 1980;106:103–10.

[32] Weber PC, Johnson JT, Myers EN. The suprahyoid approach for squamous cell carcinoma of base of the tongue. Laryngoscope 1992;102:637–40.

[33] Ariyan S. The pectoralis major myocutaneous flap. Plast Reconstr Surg 1991;117:757–66.

[34] Baek SM, Biller HF, Krespi YP, et al. The pectoralis myocutaneous island flap for reconstruction of the head and neck. Head Neck Surg 1971;47:234.

[35] Quillen CG. Latissimus dorsi myocutaneous flaps in head and neck reconstruction. Plast Reconstr Surg 1971;47:234.

[36] Netterville JL, Wood JE. The lower trapezius flap. Arch Otolaryngol Head Neck Surg 1991; 117:73–6.

[37] Urken ML, Moscoso JF, Lawson W, et al. A systematic approach to functional reconstruction of the oral cavity following partial and total glossectomy. Arch Otolaryngol Head Neck Surg 1994;120:589–601.

[38] Forastiere A, Koch W, Trotti A, et al. Head and neck cancer. N Engl J Med 2001;345: 1890–900.

[39] Hong WK, Lippman SM, Wolf GT. Recent advances in head and neck cancer-larynx preservation and chemoprevention: the Seventeenth Annual Richard Rosenthal Foundation Award Lecture. Cancer Res 1993;53:5113–20.

[40] Ward PH, Hanson DG. Reflux as an etiological factor of carcinoma of the laryngopharynx. Laryngoscope 1998;8:1195–9.

[41] Carpenter RJ, DeSanto LW, Devine KD, et al. Cancer of the hypopharynx. Arch Otolaryngol 1976;102:716–21.

[42] Feind CR. The head and neck. In: Haagensen CS, Feind CR, Herter FP, et al, editors. The lymphatics in cancer. Philadelphia: WB Saunders; 1972. p. 60.

[43] Ballantyne AJ. Significance of retropharyngeal nodes in cancer of the head and neck. Am J Surg 1964;108:500–4.

[44] Keane TJ. Carcinoma of the hypopharynx. J Otolaryngol 1982;11:227–31.

[45] Horwitz SD, Caldarelli DD, Hendrickson FR. Treatment of carcinoma of the hypopharynx. Head Neck Surg 1979;2(2):107–11.

[46] Guillamondegui OM, Meoz R, Jesse RH. Surgical treatment of squamous cell carcinoma of the pharyngeal walls. Am J Surg 1978;136:474–6.

[47] Mendenhall WM, Parsons JT, Devine JW, et al. Squamous cell carcinoma of the pyriform sinus treated with surgery and/or radiotherapy. Head Neck Surg 1987;10: 88–92.

[48] Donald PJ, Hayes HR, Dhaliwal R. Combined treatment for pyriform sinus cancer using postoperative irradiation. Otolaryngol Head Neck Surg 1980;88:738–44.

[49] Kramer S, Gelber RD, Snow JB, et al. Combined radiation therapy and surgery in the management of advanced head and neck cancer: final report of study 73–03 of the Radiation Therapy Oncology Group. Head Neck 1987;10:19–30.

[50] Ogura JH, Jurema AA, Watson RK. Partial larygopharyngectomy and neck dissection for pyriform sinus cancer. Conservation surgery with immediate reconstruction. Laryngoscope 1960;70:1399–417.

[51] Byers RM, Wolf PF, Ballantyne AJ. Rationale for elective modified neck dissection. Head Neck Surg 1988;10(3):160–7.

[52] Ogura JH, Biller HF, Wette R. Elective neck dissection for pharyngeal and laryngeal cancers: an evaluation. Ann Otol Rhinol Laryngol 1971;80:646–50.

[53] Ballantyne AJ. Principles of surgical management of cancer of the pharyngeal walls. Cancer 1967;20:663–7.

[54] Rees RS, Ivey GL, Shack RB, et al. Pectoralis major musculocutaneous flaps: long-term follow-up of hypopharyngeal reconstruction. Plast Reconstr Surg 1986;77: 586–91.

[55] Lau WF, Lam KH, Wei WI. Reconstruction of hypopharyngeal defects: do we have a choice? Am J Surg 1987;154:374–80.

[56] Coleman JJ, Searles JM, Hester TR, et al. Ten years experience with the free jejunal autograft. Am J Surg 1987;154:394–8.

[57] Harrison DF, Thompson AE. Pharyngoesophagectomy with pharyngogastric anastomosis for cancer of the hypopharynx: review of 101 operations. Head Neck Surg 1986;8: 418–28.

[58] Spector JG, Sessions DG, Emami B, et al. Squamous cell carcinoma of the pyriform sinus: a non-randomized comparison of therapeutic modalities and long-term results. Laryngoscope 1995;105:397–406.

[59] Bataini P, Brugere J, Bernier J, et al. Results of radical radiotherapeutic treatment of carcinoma of the pyriform sinus: experience of the Institut Curie. Int J Radiat Oncol Biol Phys 1982;8:1277–86.

[60] Dubois JB, Guerrier B, Di Ruggiero JM, et al. Cancer of the pyriform sinus: treatment by radiation alone and with surgery. Radiology 1986;160(3):831–6.

[61] Kraus DH, Zelefski MJ, Brock HAJ, et al. Combined surgery and radiation therapy for squamous cell carcinoma of the hypopharynx. Otolaryngol Head Neck Surg 1997;116: 637–41.

[62] Lefebvre JL, Chevalier D, Luboinski B, et al. Larynx preservation in pyriform sinus cancer: preliminary results of a European Organization for Research and Treatment of Cancer phase III study. J Natl Cancer Inst 1996;13:890–9.

[63] Beauvillain C, Mahe M, Bourdin S, et al. Final results of a randomized trial comparing chemotherapy plus radiotherapy with chemotherapy plus surgery plus radiotherapy in locally advanced resectable hypopharyngeal carcinomas. Laryngoscope 1997;107(5):648–53.

[64] Schechter GL, Wadsworth JT. Hypopharyngeal cancer. In: Bailey BB, Healy GB, Johnson JJ, et al, editors. Head and neck surgery–otolaryngology. 3rd edition. Philadelphia: Lippincott Williams & Wilkins; 2001. p. 1443–59.

[65] Denis F, Garaud P, Bardet E, et al. Final results of the 94–01 French Head and Neck Oncology and Radiotherapy Group randomized trial comparing radiotherapy alone with concomitant radiochemotherapy in advanced-stage oropharynx carcinoma. J Clin Oncol 2004;22(1):69–74.

[66] Wendt TG, Grabenbauer GG, Rodel CM, et al. Simultaneous radiochemotherapy versus radiotherapy alone in advanced head and neck cancer: a randomized multicenter study. J Clin Oncol 1998;16(4):1318–24.

[67] Brizel DM, Albers ME, Fisher SR, et al. Hyperfractionated irradiation with or without concurrent chemotherapy for locally advanced head and neck cancer. N Engl J Med 1998; 338:1798–804.

[68] Jeremic B, Shibamoto Y, Stanisavljevic B, et al. Radiation therapy alone or with concurrent low-dose daily either cisplatin or carboplatin in locally advanced unresectable squamous cell carcinoma of the head and neck: a prospective randomized trial. Radiother Oncol 1997;43: 29–37.

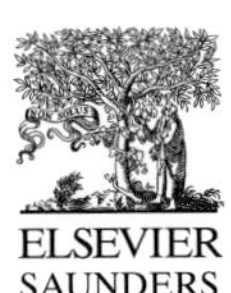

ELSEVIER
SAUNDERS

Otolaryngol Clin N Am
38 (2005) 75–85

OTOLARYNGOLOGIC
CLINICS
OF NORTH AMERICA

# Management of Cancer of the Base of Tongue

Peter Han, MD[a,*], Kenneth Hu, MD[a,b],
Douglas K. Frank, MD[a,b], Roy B. Sessions, MD[a,b],
Louis B. Harrison, MD[a,b]

[a]*Continuum Cancer Centers of New York, Beth Israel Medical Center,
St. Luke's Roosevelt Hospital, New York Eye & Ear Infirmary, New York, NY, USA*
[b]*Albert Einstein College of Medicine, New York, NY, USA*

The management of cancer of the base of tongue has improved significantly during the past decade. Currently, most patients can be treated using an organ-preservation approach that optimizes oncologic and quality-of-life outcomes. Continued advances in radiation therapy delivery and the increasing incorporation of concomitant chemotherapy into the management programs have led to excellent local control and potentially lower rates of distant metastasis. Also, the addition of a planned neck dissection has led to outstanding rates of regional control, so that some authorities question whether planned neck dissection is needed in all node-positive patients.

In this article the authors review their philosophy of management and discuss the variety of treatment options that exist. They also discuss quality-of-life outcomes, because these endpoints are essential to the optimal management of patients.

## Staging

Staging for base of tongue cancer is based on definitions given in the sixth edition of the *American Joint Committee on Cancer Cancer Staging Manual* [1]. The staging system is based on clinical examination including radiographic findings as listed in Table 1.

* Corresponding author. Department of Radiation Oncology, Beth Israel Medical Center, 10 Union Square East, Suite 4G, New York, NY 10003.
*E-mail address:* phan@bethisrael.org (P. Han).

                    *oto.theclinics.com*

## Management

There are several possible treatment strategies for base of tongue cancer. Primary radiation has replaced primary surgery as the treatment of choice in most centers, including the authors'. Primary radiation therapy allows optimization of oncologic and quality-of-life outcomes. Chemotherapy has evolved as an important part of the management strategy, especially in the presence of locoregionally advanced disease. Also, for most patients with neck disease beyond N1, planned neck dissection is often advised. Thus, a multidisciplinary approach is essential to achieve good outcomes. Radiation therapy can be administered in a variety of ways. External beam radiation therapy may be given alone or in combination with an interstitial brachytherapy boost. At Beth Israel Medical Center and St. Luke's Roosevelt Center, a planned neck dissection is performed for patients with N2–N3 disease and for select N1 patients.

The optimal scheduling and delivery of radiotherapy is not clear; good outcomes have been reported with a variety of techniques. A range of

Table 1
Staging of base of tongue cancer

| Primary tumor (T) | | Regional lymph nodes (N) | |
| --- | --- | --- | --- |
| T1 | Tumor ≤2 cm in greatest dimension | N0 | No regional lymph node |
| | | N1 | Metastasis in a single ipsilateral node, ≤3 cm in greatest dimension |
| T2 | Tumor >2 cm but not >4 cm in greatest dimension | | |
| T3 | Tumor >4 cm in greatest dimension | N2a | Metastasis in single ipsilateral node, >3 cm but ≤6 cm |
| T4a | Tumor invades the larynx, deep/extrinsic muscle of the | N2b | Metastasis in multiple ipsilateral node, ≤6 cm |
| | tongue, medial pterygoid, hard palate, or mandible | N2c | Metastasis bilateral or contralateral lymph nodes, ≤6 cm |
| T4b | Tumor invades lateral pterygoid muscle, pterygoid plates, lateral nasopharynx or skull base or encases carotid artery | N3 | Metastasis in a lymph node >6 cm |

| Distant metastasis (M) | | Stage | | | |
| --- | --- | --- | --- | --- | --- |
| M0 | No distant metastasis present | Stage 0 | Tis | N0 | M0 |
| M1 | Distant metastasis present | Stage I | T1 | N0 | M0 |
| | | Stage II | T2 | N0 | M0 |
| | | Stage III | T3 | N0 | M0 |
| | | | T1-3 | N1 | M0 |
| | | Stage IVA | T4a | N0-2 | M0 |
| | | | T1-3 | N2 | M0 |
| | | Stage IVB | T4b | Any N | M0 |
| | | | Any T | N3 | M0 |
| | | Stage IVC | Any T | Any N | M1 |

*From* Greene F, Page D, Fleming L, et al. AJCC cancer staging manual. 6th edition. New York: Springer-Verlag, 2002.

protocols using external beam radiation therapy with conventional fractionation, various hyperfractionation schemes, and the use of brachytherapy has also been studied and reported. Even among the radiation oncologists, there is still some debate regarding the optimal approach.

In our institution, the combination of external beam radiation therapy plus brachytherapy is the standard approach. Patients with T1 and T2 tumors initially receive a course of 54-Gy external beam radiation therapy using once-daily fractions of 1.8 Gy. This therapy is followed by an interstitial brachytherapy boost ranging from doses of 20 to 25 Gy delivered by a low–dose rate Iridium-192 implant. Palpable neck nodes are typically boosted using external beam radiation therapy up to 60 Gy followed by a planned neck dissection for clinically involved necks. The neck dissection is performed when the implant is placed. For T3 and T4 disease, the authors use higher doses of external beam radiation (66.6–70.2 Gy) to the primary tumor and neck with concomitant chemotherapy followed by a lower-dose implant (10–12 Gy). A planned neck dissection is still done for those with N2 or higher disease, regardless of the treatment response.

Primary surgery has been employed in various manners. Depending upon the extent of tumor, surgery may consist of partial or total glossectomy with or without a neck dissection. Typically, for more advanced disease, more extensive resections are necessary and may include supraglottic versus total pharyngo-laryngectomy with a flap reconstruction. Usually, in the presence of locally advanced disease, the patient receives postoperative external beam radiation therapy. Quality-of-life issues involving functional deficits are definitely of concern. Aside from the risks associated with surgery, the patient's ability to swallow and communicate can be compromised.

## Results

The outcomes using various modalities have been encouraging. The authors believe that the use of combined external beam irradiation plus interstitial brachytherapy has given the most consistent results in terms of local control and quality of life.

Table 2 shows the results of a number of reports of patients treated with combined external beam radiation plus interstitial brachytherapy. Local control rates of 80% to 90% for T1 through T3 disease are consistently reported, and control rates of 70% or higher for T4 disease are commonly achieved as well.

Harrison et al [2] reported on 36 patients with base of tongue primary tumors, mostly stage III or IV, treated with external beam radiation therapy and interstitial brachytherapy. Those with positive neck disease were treated with irradiation and neck dissection. The actuarial local control and survival at 2 years were 87.5%. An update with longer follow-up on 68 patients was reported [3]. At 10 years, the actuarial local controls were 87%, 93%, 82%,

Table 2
External beam radiation therapy with interstitial implant

| Study | Local control (%) | 5-year overall survival (%) | Late complications (%) |
|---|---|---|---|
| Housset [6] | | | |
| T1 | 100 | 54[a] | 10[a] |
| T2 | 74 | | |
| Harrison [2,3,23] | | | |
| T1 | 87–100 | 87[a,b] | 9–35 |
| T2 | 83–93 | | |
| T3 | 80–83 | | |
| T4 | 100 | | |
| Gibbs [5] | | | |
| T1 | 86 | Stage I/II = 43 | 17 |
| T2 | 86 | Stage III/IV = 71 | |
| T3 | 90 | | |
| T4 | 70 | | |
| Puthawala [24] | | | |
| T1 | 100 | 35[a] | 11.4 |
| T2 | 87.5 | | |
| T3 | 75 | | |
| T4 | 67 | | |
| Barrett [25] | | | |
| T1–4 | 87 | 40[a] | 20 |

[a] Includes all patients.
[b] Includes 2 year actuarial survival for all patients.
*Data from* Refs. [2,3,5,6,23–25].

and 100% for T1 to T4 disease, respectively. The 10-year actuarial local controls by nodal stage were 68%, 87%, 96%, 100%, and 100% for N0, N1, N2, N3, and NX disease, respectively. The 10-year actuarial overall survival was 57%. Goffinet et al [4] reported similar results in their series of patients treated at Stanford University. Most patients had stage III or stage IV disease. The 5-year reported actuarial survival was 70%. A recent update was published on the outcomes of 41 patients [5]. The 5-year rates of local control were 86%, 86%, 90%, and 70% for T1 to T4 disease, respectively. The 5-year overall survival rates for were 43% for stage I/II and 71% for stage III/IV disease.

One of the few series in the literature that compares outcomes using different techniques was reported by Housset et al [6]. In this series, patients with T1 and T2 disease were treated with external beam radiation therapy alone, external beam radiation therapy plus brachytherapy, or surgery plus postoperative radiation therapy. The composition of the three groups was similar, except that more patients in the group treated with external beam radiation therapy alone had purely exophytic lesions. Despite this potentially more favorable selection bias, the local failure rate was twice as high in that group. Local control in the other two groups was about 80%, demonstrating that organ-preservation therapy using external beam plus brachytherapy is feasible and does not compromise local control when compared with primary surgery.

Table 3 shows a number of reports of series that used external beam radiation therapy alone. These results are not as consistently good as those obtained external beam radiation plus brachytherapy. Some of these reports, however, show excellent outcomes, especially when hyperfractionation or accelerated fractionation is employed.

Mendenhall et al [7] reported on 217 patients treated with external beam radiation therapy alone. The majority of patients were treated with twice-daily fractionation to a mean dose of 76.8 Gy. Patients with clinically positive neck disease also underwent a planned neck dissection. A small percentage of the patients with locally advanced disease received chemotherapy. The local control rates were 96%, 91%, 81%, and 38% for T1 to T4 lesions, respectively. The overall local-regional control rate at 5 years was 72%. Absolute 5-year survival was 50% (one of two total patients), 81%, 65%, 42%, and 44% for stage I, II, III, IVa, and IVb disease, respectively. In their discussion, the authors compared their outcomes with published reports using external beam radiation therapy with or without brachytherapy or with definitive surgery with or without adjuvant radiation therapy. They found that surgery has no obvious advantage over radiation therapy, including quality-of-life outcomes. As listed in Table 3, the local control rates with external beam radiation therapy are promising, but the data seem to be inconsistent.

Surgery has resulted in local control rates ranging from 75% to 85%. Kraus et al [8] reported a 5-year overall survival rate of 66% in patients with T1 and T2 disease treated with definitive surgery. Some patients in this study received postoperative radiation therapy. In this series, which also included locoregionally advanced tumors, the local control rate was 82%. Weber et al [9] report a similar local control rate of 83% for early primary tumors. They also report that exophytic tumors have a higher primary control rate, 84%, versus 58% for ulcerative-infiltrative tumors.

Given these data, the authors' preference is to use combined external beam radiation therapy plus brachytherapy as the definitive management of the primary site. Of course, treatment must always be individualized, and all options must be considered. Also, it is certainly clear that, in experienced hands, good results can be achieved using other approaches.

## Organ-preservation therapy using concomitant radiation and chemotherapy

Several overviews have reported the potential benefit of adding chemotherapy to radiation [10–12]. Pignon et al [10] performed a large meta-analysis examining the benefit of chemotherapy with definitive radiation therapy for squamous cell carcinoma of the head and neck. There was an overall pooled hazard ratio of death of 0.90 with $P < 0.0001$ in favor of chemotherapy, corresponding to an absolute survival benefit of 4% at 2 and

Table 3
Results using external beam radiation therapy only

| Study | Local control (%) | 5-year overall survival (%) | Late complications (%) |
| --- | --- | --- | --- |
| Housset[a] [6] | | | |
| T1 | 79 | 17[b] | 10 |
| T2 | 47 | | |
| Jaulerry[a] [26] | | | |
| T1 | 96 | 49 | NR |
| T2 | 57 | 29 | |
| T3 | 45 | 23 | |
| T4 | 23 | 16 | |
| Brunin[a] [27] | | | |
| T1 | 83 | Stage I = 53 | NR |
| T2 | 54 | Stage II/III = 34 | |
| T3 | 38 | Stage IV = 18 | |
| T4 | 18 | | |
| Fein[c,d] [28] | | | |
| T1 | 90 | Stage I = 45 | 3 |
| T2 | 92 | Stage II = 61 | |
| T3 | 73 | Stage III = 60 | |
| T4 | 35 | Stage IVA/B = 40/25 | |
| Mendenhall[c] [7] | | | |
| T1 | 96 | Stage I = 50[e] | 3.7 |
| T2 | 91 | Stage II = 81 | |
| T3 | 81 | Stage III = 65 | |
| T4 | 38 | Stage IVA = 42 | |
| | | Stage IVB = 44 | |

*Abbreviations:* NR, not reported.
[a] Includes only once-daily fractionation.
[b] Includes both T1–2 patients.
[c] Includes both once-daily and twice-daily fractionations.
[d] Includes all of the oropharyngeal sites.
[e] Includes total of only two patients.
*Data from* Refs. [6,7,26–28].

5 years. In addition, there was a significant benefit with concomitant chemotherapy, whereas adjuvant or neoadjuvant chemotherapy failed to demonstrate any advantage.

A French Head and Neck Oncology and Radiotherapy Group reported on a randomized trial for locally advanced oropharyngeal carcinoma with base of tongue primary tumors in 37% of the patient population [13]. The patients were randomly assigned to treatment with radiation therapy alone (70 Gy in 35 fractions) or concomitant radiation with carboplatin (daily bolus of 70 mg/m$^2$/day) and 5-fluorouracil (continuous infusion of 600 mg/m$^2$/day), for 4 days every 3 weeks, for three cycles, with an identical radiation protocol. With a median follow up of 5.5 years, there was a significant 5-year overall survival benefit in favor of combined therapy versus radiation alone (22.4% versus 15.8%, respectively). In addition, there was a significant improvement in 5-year specific disease-free survival (26.6% versus 14.6%, respectively) and locoregional control (47.6% versus 24.7%, respectively). Despite more aggressive therapy, failure occurred at the primary tumor site in 65% of the patients relapsing after combined-modality treatment. These patients fared much worse than did patients in other series already discussed.

Given these emerging data supporting the benefit of concomitant chemotherapy (Table 4), the authors' treatment paradigm has evolved to use concomitant chemotherapy for most patients with stage III or stage IV disease. Although one could debate whether a patient with T1-2N1M0 disease would benefit, the authors' practice has certainly evolved to include concomitant chemotherapy for the majority of patients with T3 to T4 disease, or N2 or higher neck disease. Also, because the data in the organ-preservation context are most supportive of cisplatin-based chemotherapy

Table 4
Randomized external beam radiation therapy and chemotherapy trials

| Study | Patients enrolled | Local control (%) | 3-year overall survival (%) | Severe late toxicity (%) |
|---|---|---|---|---|
| Brizel [29] | | | | |
|   HF RT alone | 122 | 44 | 34 | 9 |
|   C+HF RT | | 70 | 55 | 11 |
|     (Cisplatin/5FU) | | ($P = 0.08$) | (p = 0.07) | (not significant) |
| Wendt [30] | | | | |
|   RT alone | 298 | 17 | 24 | 6.4 |
|   C+RT | | 36 | 48 | 10 |
|     (cisplatin/5-FU/LV) | | ($P < 0.004$) | (p < 0.003) | (not significant) |
| Adelstein [31] | | | | |
|   RT alone | 295 | NR | 23 | 51[a] |
|   C+RT | | | 37[b] | 85[c] |
|     (cisplatin) | | | | |
|   C+split-RT | | | 27 | 72[d] |
|     (5-FU, cisplatin) | | | | |
| GORTEC [13][e] | | | | |
|   RT alone | 226 | 24.7 | 15.8[f] | 1.2[g] |
|   C+RT | | 47.6 | 22.4 | 2.0 |
|     (carboplatin/5FU) | | ($P = 0.002$) | ($P = 0.05$) | (not significant) |

*Abbreviations:* C, chemotherapy; HF, hyperfractionated; LV, leucovorin; RT, radiation therapy; 5-FU, 5-fluorouracil.

NR = Not reported.

[a] Grade 3–5 acute toxicity. Late toxicity were not reported.

[b] The $P = 0.014$ between arms one and two.

[c] The $P < 0.0001$ between arms one and two.

[d] The $P < 0.001$ between arms one and three.

[e] Only oropharyngeal primaries tumor were eligible.

[f] Reported 5 year overall survival.

[g] Grade 4 only.

*Data from* Refs. [13,29–31].

[14], the authors tend to favor the use of cisplatin unless the patient is enrolled in a clinical trial evaluating other drug combinations.


## Planned neck dissection

Patients who have neck recurrences typically have poor outcomes. To increase neck control, many have endorsed the practice of a planned neck dissection after external beam radiation therapy in patients with advanced neck metastases. Mendenhall et al [15] reported the University of Florida experience in planned neck dissection after irradiation and concluded that regional control of advanced neck disease increases with the addition of a planned dissection.

Frank et al [16] reviewed the Beth Israel experience with planned neck dissection. He analyzed 51 planned neck dissections in 39 patients who had undergone definitive chemoradiotherapy for locoregionally advanced head and neck cancer. Patients received a mean dose of 67 Gy to the primary tumor and 62.5 Gy to the involved nodal disease. After a mean follow up of 18 months, there has been only one neck recurrence. This occurred in a patient with N2a disease. There were no neck recurrences in the 41 dissected necks of patents undergoing modified and selective neck dissection procedures. Eighteen neck specimens were found to have residual carcinoma present, but only one patient had a neck recurrence. In addition, the clinical absence of residual disease after the chemoradiation therapy did not always predict a complete pathologic response. The surgery was well tolerated, with only two limited surgical complications. Brizel et al [17] recently reported an analysis of adjuvant neck dissection after concurrent chemoradiation for advanced head and neck disease. The 4-year disease-free survival rate was 75% for patients with N2 and N3 disease who had a clinical complete response and underwent modified neck dissection, versus 53% for patients who had a clinical complete response but did not undergo modified neck dissection ($P = 0.08$). The 4-year overall survival rates were 77% and 50%, respectively, for these two groups of patients ($P = 0.04$). There seemed to be no difference in outcome for N1 disease, irrespective of clinical response or the addition of a neck dissection. Newkirk et al [18] noted only two failures in the neck out of 40 neck dissections in 33 patients after organ-preservation therapy and planned neck dissection. Analysis by McHamm et al [19] of 109 patients with N2 and N3 disease after definitive chemoradiation therapy and planned neck dissection showed that clinical response alone is not a good predictor of pathologic outcome of planned neck dissection. Thus, the difficulty with clinical assessment, plus the excellent regional control, supports the continued use of planned neck dissection after organ-preservation therapy in patients with disease beyond N1. Time will tell whether emerging data using positron emission tomography (PET) scans or PET/CT will allow to more accurate predictions as to which patients require planned neck dissection.

## Quality of life

Harrison et al [20] reported on the quality-of-life issues and performance status in base of tongue cancer patients treated with external beam radiation therapy with brachytherapy boost versus primary surgery. A Performance Status Scale for Head and Neck Cancer (PSS) developed by List et al [21] was used for the assessment. This scale, scored from 0 to 100, evaluated the three basic functions of eating in public, understandable speech, and normalcy of diet. For eating in public, patients with T1 and T2 tumors had a score of 85 versus 75 ($P = 0.31$), and patients with T3 and T4 disease had a score of 82 versus 35 ($P < 0.001$) for radiation versus surgery, respectively. For understandable speech, patients with T1 and T2 disease had scores of 92 versus 65 ($P = 0.0021$), and patients with T3 and T4 disease had scores of 95 versus 35 ($P < 0.0001$) for radiation versus surgery, respectively. For normalcy of diet, patients with T1 and T2 disease had scores of 74 versus 50 ($P = 0.047$), and patients with T3 and T4 disease had scores of 78 versus 32 ($P = 0.0012$) for radiation versus surgery, respectively. These data indicate that there is a functional and quality-of-life benefit to primary radiation therapy. In addition, other quality-of-life measures, such as the ability to return to work and maintain income, show favorable outcomes with primary radiation [22]. The major quality-of-life issues in these patients include xerostomia and potential difficulty in swallowing. Efforts are under way to attempt to minimize these long-term quality-of-life issues.

## Summary

In the management of base of tongue cancer, multidisciplinary care and combined modality therapy can lead to better functional and oncologic outcomes. Although the care of every patient should be individualized, most patients are candidates for organ-preservation therapy that can optimize both cure rates and patients' quality of life.

## References


[1] Greene F, Page D, Fleming I, et al. American Joing Committee on Cancer cancer staging manual. 6th edition. New York: Springer-Verlag; 2002.

[2] Harrison LB, Zelefsky MJ, Sessions RB, et al. Base-of-tongue cancer treated with external beam irradiation plus brachytherapy: oncologic and functional outcome. Radiology 1992; 184(1):267–70.

[3] Harrison LB, Lee HJ, Pfister DG, et al. Long term results of primary radiotherapy with/without neck dissection for squamous cell cancer of the base of tongue. Head Neck 1998; 20(8):668–73.

[4] Goffinet DR, Fee WE Jr, Wells J, et al. 192-Ir pharyngoepiglottic fold interstitial implants. The key to successful treatment of base tongue carcinoma by radiation therapy. Cancer 1985; 55(5):941–8.

[5] Gibbs IC, Le QT, Shah RD, et al. Long-term outcomes after external beam irradiation and brachytherapy boost for base-of-tongue cancers. Int J Radiat Oncol Biol Phys 2003;57(2): 489–94.

[6] Housset M, Baillet F, Dessard-Diana B, et al. A retrospective study of three treatment techniques for T1–T2 base of tongue lesions: surgery plus postoperative radiation, external radiation plus interstitial implantation and external radiation alone. Int J Radiat Oncol Biol Phys 1987;13(4):511–6.

[7] Mendenhall WM, Stringer SP, Amdur RJ, et al. Is radiation therapy a preferred alternative to surgery for squamous cell carcinoma of the base of tongue? J Clin Oncol 2000;18(1):35–42.

[8] Kraus DH, Vastola AP, Huvos AG, et al. Surgical management of squamous cell carcinoma of the base of the tongue. Am J Surg 1993;166(4):384–8.

[9] Weber RS, Gidley P, Morrison WH, et al. Treatment selection for carcinoma of the base of the tongue. Am J Surg 1990;160(4):415–9.

[10] Pignon JP, Bourhis J, Domenge C, et al. Chemotherapy added to locoregional treatment for head and neck squamous-cell carcinoma: three meta-analyses of updated individual data. MACH-NC [Meta-Analysis of Chemotherapy on Head and Neck Cancer] Collaborative Group. Lancet 2000;18;355(9208):949–55.

[11] Munro AJ. An overview of randomised controlled trials of adjuvant chemotherapy in head and neck cancer. Br J Cancer 1995;71(1):83–91.

[12] Bourhis J, Eschwege F. Radiotherapy-chemotherapy combinations in head and neck squamous cell carcinoma: overview of randomized trials. Anticancer Res 1996;16(4C):2397–402.

[13] Denis F, Garaud P, Bardet E, et al. Final results of the 94–01 French Head and Neck Oncology and Radiotherapy Group randomized trial comparing radiotherapy alone with concomitant radiochemotherapy in advanced-stage oropharynx carcinoma. J Clin Oncol 2004;22(1):69–76.

[14] Forastiere AA, Goepfert H, Maor M, et al. Concurrent chemotherapy and radiotherapy for organ preservation in advanced laryngeal cancer. N Engl J Med 2003;349(22):2091–8.

[15] Mendenhall WM, Villaret DB, Amdur RJ, et al. Planned neck dissection after definitive radiotherapy for squamous cell carcinoma of the head and neck. Head Neck 2002;24(11): 1012–8.

[16] Frank DK, Hu K, Culliney B, et al. planned neck dissection after concomitant radio-chemotherapy for advanced head and neck cancer [abstract #s322]. Presented at the 6th International Conference on Head and Neck Cancer. Washington, DC, August 7–11, 2004.

[17] Brizel DM, Prosnitz RG, Hunter S, et al. Necessity for adjuvant neck dissection in setting of concurrent chemoradiation for advanced head-and-neck cancer. Int J Radiat Oncol Biol Phys 2004;58(5):1418–23.

[18] Newkirk KA, Cullen KJ, Harter KW, et al. Planned neck dissection for advanced primary head and neck malignancy treated with organ preservation therapy: disease control and survival outcomes. Head Neck 2001;23(2):73–9.

[19] McHam SA, Adelstein DJ, Rybicki LA, et al. Who merits a neck dissection after definitive chemoradiotherapy for N2–N3 squamous cell head and neck cancer? Head Neck 2003; 25(10):791–8.

[20] Harrison LB, Zelefsky MJ, Armstrong JG, et al. Performance status after treatment for squamous cell cancer of the base of tongue—a comparison of primary radiation therapy versus primary surgery. Int J Radiat Oncol Biol Phys 1994;30(4):953–7.

[21] List MA, Ritter-Sterr C, Lansky SB. A performance status scale for head and neck cancer patients. Cancer 1990;1;66(3):564–9.

[22] Harrison LB, Zelefsky MJ, Pfister DG, et al. Detailed quality of life assessment in patients treated with primary radiotherapy for squamous cell cancer of the base of the tongue. Head Neck 1997;19(3):169–75.

[23] Harrison LB, Sessions RB, Strong EW, et al. Brachytherapy as part of the definitive management of squamous cancer of the base of tongue. Int J Radiat Oncol Biol Phys 1989; 17(6):1309–12.

[24] Puthawala AA, Syed AM, Eads DL, et al. Limited external beam and interstitial 192-iridium irradiation in the treatment of carcinoma of the base of the tongue: a ten year experience. Int J Radiat Oncol Biol Phys 1988;14(5):839–48.

[25] Barrett WL, Gleich L, Wilson K, et al. Organ preservation with interstitial radiation for base of tongue cancer. Am J Clin Oncol 2002;25(5):485–8.

[26] Jaulerry C, Rodriguez J, Brunin F, et al. Results of radiation therapy in carcinoma of the base of the tongue. The Curie Institute experience with about 166 cases. Cancer 1991;67(6): 1532–8.

[27] Brunin F, Mosseri V, Jaulerry C, et al. Cancer of the base of the tongue: past and future. Head Neck 1999;21(8):751–9.

[28] Fein DA, Lee WR, Amos WR, et al. Oropharyngeal carcinoma treated with radiotherapy: a 30-year experience. Int J Radiat Oncol Biol Phys 1996;34(2):289–96.

[29] Brizel DM, Albers ME, Fisher SR, et al. Hyperfractionated irradiation with or without concurrent chemotherapy for locally advanced head and neck cancer. N Engl J Med 1998; 338(25):1798–804.

[30] Wendt TG, Grabenbauer GG, Rodel CM, et al. Simultaneous radiochemotherapy versus radiotherapy alone in advanced head and neck cancer: a randomized multicenter study. J Clin Oncol 1998;16(4):1318–24.

[31] Adelstein DJ, Li Y, Adams GL, et al. An intergroup phase III comparison of standard radiation therapy and two schedules of concurrent chemoradiotherapy in patients with unresectable squamous cell head and neck cancer. J Clin Oncol 2003;21(1):92–8.

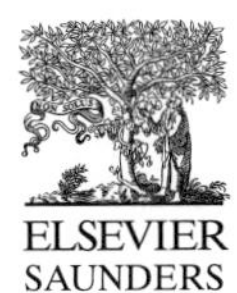

Otolaryngol Clin N Am
38 (2005) 87–97

OTOLARYNGOLOGIC
CLINICS
OF NORTH AMERICA

# Evaluation and Management of Malignant Cervical Lymphadenopathy with an Unknown Primary Tumor

Elizabeth J. Mahoney, MD,
Jeffrey H. Spiegel, MD, FACS*

*Department of Otolaryngology-Head and Neck Surgery,
Boston University School of Medicine, 88 East Newton Street,
Suite D-616, Boston, MA 02118, USA*

Periodically physicians involved in the management of head and neck cancer encounter a patient with biopsy-demonstrated carcinoma within a cervical lymph node but with no clinically detectable primary tumor site within the upper aerodigestive tract. Presumed metastatic carcinoma within cervical lymph nodes with an unknown primary site is relatively rare, representing only 3% to 5% of all head and neck cancers [1]. Explanations for this phenomenon are speculative, and although the roles of panendoscopy (directed laryngoscopy, esophagoscopy, bronchoscopy) and directed biopsies are generally accepted, many questions about how to employ and interpret new radiographic technologies and about appropriate management remain unanswered.

This article reviews current information regarding the diagnostic evaluation of the patient with malignant cervical disease with an unknown primary tumor site, prognostic indicators for these patients, and treatment strategies.

## Etiology

Carcinoma metastatic to the neck with an unknown primary tumor site accounts for approximately 3% to 5% of all head and neck cancers. Most patients with metastatic cervical adenopathy have squamous cell carcinoma

* Corresponding author.
*E-mail address:* Jeffrey.Spiegel@bmc.org (J.H. Spiegel).



*oto.theclinics.com*

or poorly differentiated carcinoma. Adenocarcinoma is rarely identified within a metastatic node; in these cases, attention should focus on disease below the clavicles, including the lung and breast. The otolaryngologist should exclude disease in the salivary glands, sinuses, thyroid, and parathyroid glands. The remainder of this discussion focuses on the evaluation and management of patients with squamous cell carcinoma or undifferentiated carcinoma metastatic to the neck with an unknown primary site.

It has been hypothesized that the patient with malignant cervical lymphadenopathy but unknown primary site may in fact have no upper aerodigestive tract primary site. Rather, the tumor primarily developed in the neck within squamous cells remaining as remnants of branchial cleft cysts. Although this theory is intriguing, little evidence has been presented to support it, and it has largely fallen out of favor. Others have suggested that these patients have exhibited spontaneous regression of the primary tumor site with persistence of cervical metastases. Unfortunately, there is no evidence for the spontaneous regression of squamous cell carcinoma [2]. As a result, this theory, too, has not taken hold. Improvements in radiographic technologies have occasionally allowed the detection of primary sites in patients who were previously considered to have unknown primary tumors. Similarly, the addition of directed biopsies (including tonsillectomy) during panendoscopy in the evaluation of these patients has allowed a small upper aerodigestive tract malignant focus to be identified in some patients with presumed unknown primary sites. Current theory is that unknown primary tumors are likely to be primary tumors that exist in the upper aerodigestive tracts or skin but are subclinical at the time of presentation. Thus unknown primary tumors remain undetected but are presumed to be present. Anecdotal support of this theory includes the identification of some primary tumors during or after treatment. On more than one occasion, the senior author on this paper has had a patient with unknown primary tumor who develops an area of early mucosal change after the initial part of radiation therapy. Biopsy of these areas may help localize the primary site. In other patients, small primary sites may be eliminated by radiation therapy. Thus, although a cervical metastasis can truly be labeled as a metastasis with an unknown primary tumor only after an exhaustive diagnostic work-up, it seems likely that for each of these patients there is, in fact, a primary tumor site that cannot be identified by current methods.

**Diagnostic evaluation**

Clearly, in all patients categorized as having an unknown primary tumor, a neck mass has been identified at some point. The evaluation of a neck mass is well known to the otolaryngologist and is not reviewed here. The physician should perform a careful office examination of the upper aerodigestive tract as part of a thorough history and physical examination. Only after this examination has failed to identify any suspicious sites can the patient be tentatively classified as having an unknown primary tumor.

To stratify risks and help direct the search, any history of tobacco or alcohol use should be ascertained. Also important is a history of sun exposure, because squamous cell carcinoma of the skin and scalp may present with a metastatic node. Signs and symptoms not limited to but including otalgia, hoarseness, dysphagia, weight loss, and trismus should be specifically elicited. Physical examination should typically include palpation of the tonsillar fossae and base of tongue as well as flexible nasopharyngoscopy. On examination of the neck, careful attention should be paid to the size and extent of adenopathy, cranial nerve deficits, and fixation of nodes to surrounding structures or skin.

Epstein-Barr virus serologies have also been proposed as a minimally invasive test that can provide additional evidence for a nasopharyngeal primary tumor [2], although careful examination of the nasopharynx through flexible fiberoptic endoscopy and directed biopsies of the nasopharynx are considered higher yield. Finally, fine-needle aspiration (FNA) of a suspicious cervical node should be performed if a patient is referred without prior histopathologic evaluation. FNA is preferred to open biopsy because it is easily performed, has little morbidity, and is less likely to seed tumor cells along the tract [3].

The character and location of neck nodes may provide important information regarding the site of the primary tumor. Supraclavicular nodes, for example, are more likely to be associated with a primary site below the level of the clavicles, such as the breast or lung [4]. In the case of squamous cell carcinoma with occult primary tumor, the jugulodigastric or upper jugular nodes are most frequently involved. These nodal basins typically provide primary drainage for the soft palate, tonsil, base of tongue, pyriform sinus, and supraglottic larynx. The middle jugular nodes provide primary drainage for the supraglottic larynx, inferior pyriform sinus, and postcricoid region. The most inferior jugular nodes receive drainage from the thyroid, trachea, and cervical esophagus. Posterior triangle adenopathy may point to a nasopharyngeal primary tumor.

Preoperative diagnostic evaluation is not complete without imaging. Contrast-enhanced CT from the skull base to the level of the thoracic inlet is indicated. Chest radiographs or extension of the CT scan through the thorax should be performed to assess for a primary lung tumor. Other recommendations include a metabolic profile with liver function testing and consideration of abdominal CT for proper staging. The neck CT is important in the search for an occult primary site and also to evaluate the extent of nodal disease, check for obvious extracapsular spread and soft-tissue involvement, and examine for suspicious nodes in the contralateral neck [5].

Recently, attention has focused on the use of fluorodeoxyglucose–positron emission tomography (FDG-PET) as an adjunct in the diagnostic evaluation for an unknown primary tumor. Although the usefulness of PET scanning is still evolving, many practitioners now incorporate this imaging study in their diagnostic evaluation for an occult primary tumor. Tumor cells have a higher metabolic rate than normal tissue; head and neck neoplasms have an increased glycolytic rate. Thus, head and neck neoplasms are good candidates for metabolic imaging and can be traced using a glucose analogue, 2-[fluorine-18]fluoro-2-deoxy-D-glucose. FDG uptake reflects cellular metabolism, and cellular processes such as infection, neoplasm, or inflammation are characterized by increased metabolic activity and consequent accumulation of the FDG tracer [6]. This accumulation, which appears as a "hot" spot on PET imaging, may help locate an unknown primary tumor.

In a small 1999 study, Aasar et al [6] demonstrated that the addition of FDG-PET to the diagnostic evaluation for unknown primary tumors of the head and neck detected two primary tumors not detected on physical examination or with traditional CT or MRI. A subsequent Danish study demonstrated that FDG PET detected a primary tumor in 24% of patients with metastatic cervical adenopathy and otherwise negative clinical and radiologic evaluation [7]. A key limitation of PET has been the size of tumor it can detect. Commonly available PET scanners may have a resolution of approximately 1 cm. That is, they will inconsistently detect lesions smaller than this size. Of course, for the majority of tumors, a 1 cm lesion will be quite evident on both physical examination and CT or MRI. Newer-generation PET scanners are halving this resolution to approximately 5 mm. It is reasonable to expect that with time the size resolution of these machines will continue to improve.

An additional limitation of PET scanning has been the anatomically nonspecific image produced by these scanners. Hot spots appear as general regions without good borders, so whereas it may be possible to state that the left side of the base of tongue appears "hot," any additional information regarding size or localization would be inaccurate. Newer scanners that supplement PET with CT fusion techniques are becoming available. These machines can overlay the images so that the hot areas are visible as colored halos over the CT scan image, greatly facilitating the accuracy and localization of the PET technology. With improving resolution, improving markers, and combination technology such as PET/CT, it is expected that this technology can significantly improve the ability to identify the origin of malignant cervical lymphadenopathy with an unknown primary site. PET/CT may in the future change the radiographic evaluation of neck disease as well, because small (<1 cm) nodes that are considered not suspicious on CT could be shown to be likely malignant if they "glow" on PET/CT [8] (Figs. 1 and 2).

Along with improving resolution and fusing PET images with CT, PET technology will probably be improved by the development of new and specific tracers. These new materials may more specifically select malignant

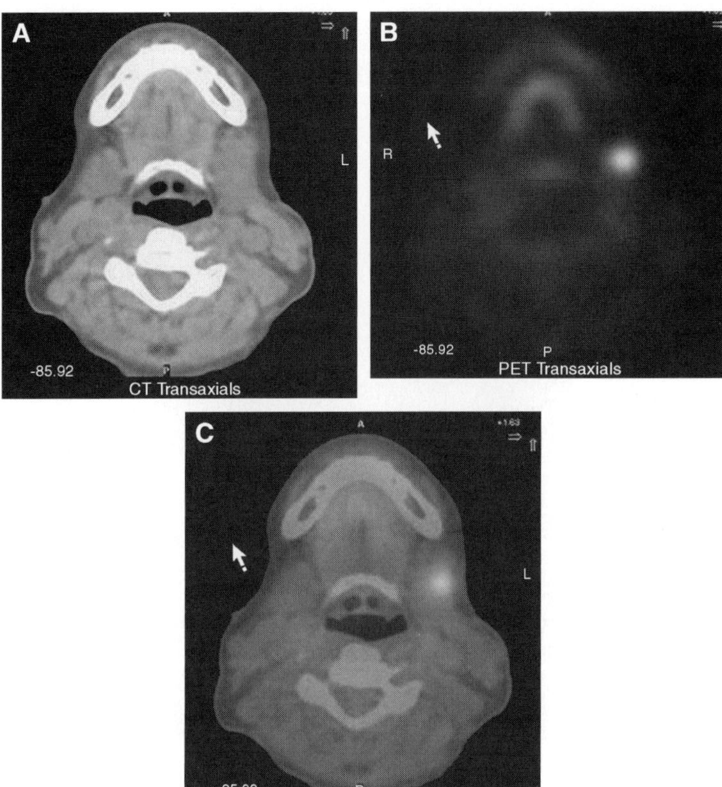

Fig. 1. Case 1. Patient with left submandibular mass, but unknown primary tumor. (*A*) Mass on CT. (*B*) Mass enhancing on PET scan. (*C*) Overlay provides most useful information on PET-CT image. (Courtesy of Osamu Sakai, MD, PhD, and Nirav P. Shah, MD, Department of Radiology, Boston Medical Center, Boston, MA.)

cells, thus reducing the rate of false positivity that is seen in inflammation and in some common tissues (eg, kidneys, bladder). Imaging, regardless of modality, should precede endoscopy with biopsy so that suspicious areas can be adequately addressed through directed biopsy and to ensure that postoperative edema does not compromise interpretation of the imaging study. To summarize, at present, most available reports suggest that PET scanning may provide some diagnostic localization benefit in the evaluation of the patient with the unknown primary tumor site, but it is not reliable and perhaps not cost effective. Thus, PET scanning should not currently be considered a necessary part of the evaluation of these patients.

Evaluation of a cervical metastasis with an unidentified primary site typically involves panendoscopy under anesthesia with directed biopsies. Panendoscopy is usually regarded as including direct laryngoscopy, rigid cervical esophagoscopy, bronchoscopy, and an examination of the nasopharynx by palpation or an endoscope. If no primary lesion is

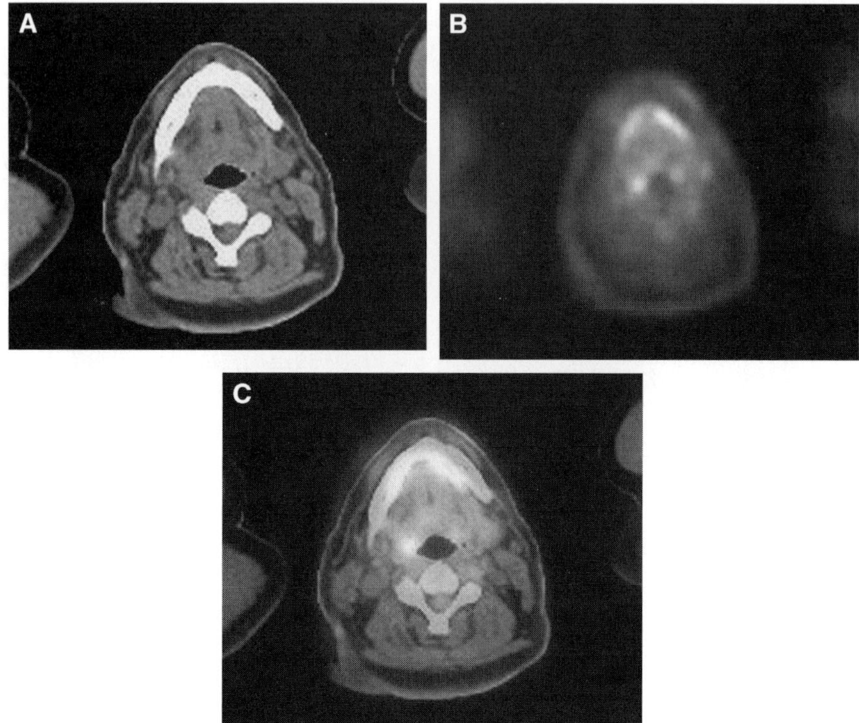

Fig. 2. Case 2. Patient with malignant neck node. These images obtained in evaluation for primary site. (*A*) CT. (*B*) Enhancement on PET scan. (*C*) Enhancement localized to tonsil on PET-CT. (Courtesy of Osamu Sakai, MD, PhD, and Nirav P. Shah, MD, Department of Radiology, Boston Medical Center, Boston, MA.)

identified, directed biopsies are then taken. The consensus in the literature is that directed biopsies should include the nasopharynx, tonsils, pyriform sinus, hypopharynx, postcricoid region, and base of tongue. Previous studies suggested that the most common sites of primary tumor detected on panendoscopy were the nasopharynx and hypopharynx. With the advent of flexible fiberoptic endoscopy, these primary sites are now often detected at the time of the initial physical examination. In a recent University of Florida study, the most common sites of primary cancer detected at the time of panendoscopy under general anesthesia seem now to have shifted to include the tonsillar fossa or base of tongue, whereas previous reports found the nasopharynx and hypopharynx to be the most common sites of primary tumor [9].

Because the tonsil remains a common site of primary tumor, most clinicians advocate tonsillectomy in addition to directed biopsies in the work-up of an unknown primary tumor. Questions regarding whether random tonsil biopsies or tonsillectomy should be performed in the evaluation of an unknown primary site and whether such tonsillectomy should be ipsilateral or bilateral tonsillectomy continue to be controversial. In a 1998 study at Johns Hopkins Hospital, McQuone et al [10] demonstrated that the detection rate of occult tonsillar carcinoma is increased by performing tonsillectomy rather than focal tonsillar biopsy. Although only 13% of tonsillar biopsy specimens were positive for squamous cell carcinoma, 39% of the patients undergoing bilateral tonsillectomy for work-up of an unknown primary site were found to have squamous cell carcinoma within a tonsil. Furthermore, one patient was found to have squamous cell carcinoma in both tonsils, strengthening the argument for bilateral tonsillectomy. In addition to identifying the rare case of bilateral or contralateral squamous cell carcinoma within tonsillar specimens, many clinicians prefer bilateral tonsillectomy for practical reasons. Bilateral tonsillectomy does not significantly increase the morbidity associated with unilateral tonsillectomy and eliminates the asymmetry that can confound follow-up examination after a unilateral procedure [5].

## Treatment

In the otolaryngologist's armamentarium, several different treatment strategies are available for the management of the true unknown primary site and squamous cell carcinoma metastatic to the neck. Whether radiation therapy is sufficient treatment for control of neck disease and whether potential primary sites should be irradiated or simply followed are controversial. Additional controversy focuses on whether radiation should be offered to patients pre- or postoperatively. Finally, questions have surfaced about whether the contralateral neck needs to be treated. Which treatment strategy provides the best outcome remains a subject of debate in the literature.

In discussing treatment strategies, it is important first to have an understanding of prognostic factors. In all large series, lymph nodal stage has correlated with outcome. As highlighted earlier, supraclavicular lymph node metastases are more likely to be associated with disease below the clavicles, and, hence, are associated with poorer survival. Histologic extracapsular spread has been noted to affect survival adversely in most large series as well. Some studies have also suggested that discovery of a primary tumor worsens prognosis; however, several large studies including a large 1990 M.D. Anderson study have found no correlation between outcome and subsequent identification of a primary site [2]. As might be expected, more primary sites were identified in patients treated with surgery than in patients treated with radiation. Although treatment protocols may vary by institution and clinician bias, there is a consensus that advanced nodal disease and extracapsular spread necessitate more aggressive therapy [11,12].

For the sake of completeness, a review of nodal staging is provided here. N1 disease is a single ipsilateral node less than 3 cm. A single ipsilateral node larger than 3 cm but not more than 6 cm is classified as N2a disease. The N2b subclassification refers to multiple ipsilateral nodes, none greater than 6 cm, and N2c includes metastases in bilateral or contralateral nodes, none greater than 6 cm. N3 disease involves a lymph node larger than 6 cm.

For the few patients presenting with N1 or N2a disease, single-modality therapy is a reasonable approach. Acceptable courses of treatment include neck dissection alone, radiation alone, and neck dissection plus radiation if extracapsular spread is noted on histopathologic analysis. A 1998 review from M.D. Anderson recommends that patients with N1 or small mobile N2a disease be treated with neck dissection alone and that postoperative radiation therapy be reserved for cases of extracapsular spread, multiple nodes, or connective tissue invasion [11]. The 5-year disease-specific survival rates were 85% in patients with a solitary node and 58% in patients with multiple nodes. Mendenhall et al [9] agree that patients with a solitary positive neck node may be treated with neck dissection alone unless multiple positive nodes are noted on exploration or extracapsular extension is seen on histologic analysis. Similarly, in patients who have undergone an excisional biopsy of a solitary node before referral, the neck may be treated with radiation alone with a 95% likelihood of neck control [11]. Weir et al [13] similarly found an 88% control rate for 63 patients given radiation alone after excisional biopsy of a single node. Thus, single-modality therapy in patients with N1 and N2a disease is reasonable. For patients with disease beyond N1 or N2a, combined modality therapy is recommended.

Patients with more advanced disease, in contrast, are triaged into an arm of treatment that includes both surgery and radiotherapy. The timing of radiation therapy also is a source of controversy. Proponents of pre-operative radiation therapy argue that surgical complications do not delay the initiation of radiotherapy, target tissues are theoretically better oxygenated in the preoperative state, and radioresistant primary tumors may become evident over the course of radiation therapy and can be removed with one definitive surgical procedure if radiation therapy is implemented before the planned neck dissection [5]. Proponents of postoperative radiation therapy argue that a neck dissection before radiotherapy allows improved delineation of disease extent and better staging through pathologic evaluation of the neck dissection specimen [13]. Although adjuvant chemotherapy has shown mixed results, it is often recommended in cases of inoperable disease or with distant metastases. There is also some evidence that concurrent chemotherapy and radiotherapy in the postoperative setting improve locoregional control rates.

The decision to include suspected primary sites in the radiation field also remains controversial. Certainly, the challenge facing clinicians is deciding how to maximize the chance of survival while minimizing treatment morbidity. Review of the literature reveals a trend toward treating both the ipsilateral and contralateral necks as well as potential mucosal primary sites. Certainly, many of the potential primary sites (ie, base of tongue, nasopharynx, supraglottis) are known for their propensity for bilateral nodal drainage. In a study including postoperative radiation to potential primary mucosal sites, Davidson et al [12] describe improved control of neck disease in patients treated with combined-modality therapy; this improved control of neck disease, however, did not translate into improvement in overall survival. Studies have shown a significant decrease in the number of primary tumors identified in patients treated with mucosal irradiation, but, again, this decrease has not translated into a survival advantage [14]. Nonetheless, Tong et al [14] point out that treatment limited to the involved side of the neck alone may compromise further radiation therapy should a primary mucosal site emerge. For this reason, bilateral radiation to the neck and mucosal sites is recommended.

Debate continues to center around which portals should be included in the radiation therapy. The consensus seems to be that the oral cavity and a laryngeal strip can be excluded, but the base of tongue, hypopharynx, and supraglottic sites should be included [15]. The decision to include the nasopharynx should be based on whether metastases are high and posterior and whether demographic factors suggest that the patient is at high risk for a nasopharyngeal primary site [12]. Sparing of the oral cavity and of an anterior strip approximating the anterior true vocal cords may significantly decrease the morbidity of the mucosal irradiation.

Regarding ipsilateral versus bilateral treatment of the sides of the neck, Carlson et al [16] demonstrated that the rates of local control for ipsilateral and bilateral neck irradiation were 53% and 90%, respectively. Reddy et al [17] also reported a series comparing ipsilateral radiotherapy with radiation delivered to both sides of the neck and sites of mucosal primaries. Significantly better neck control was demonstrated in the group receiving radiation to both sides of the neck and mucosal sites. The identification of a mucosal primary lesion was also significantly higher in the group receiving radiation only to the ipsilateral neck.

Finally, recent discussion has focused on the extent of neck dissection indicated in the patient with a cervical metastasis and unknown primary lesion. A growing body of evidence suggests that a selective neck dissection including the involved level and contiguous levels with appropriate sacrifice of involved structures is reasonable. Appropriate use of selective neck dissection can minimize the postoperative morbidity associated with modified or radical neck dissection without compromising neck control and survival [18].

Even with advances in treatment protocols, the overall 5-year survival for squamous cell carcinoma metastatic to a cervical node with an unknown primary site remains approximately 50%. The 2-, 5-, and 10-year actuarial disease-specific survival rates have been reported to be 82%, 74%, and 68%, respectively; the overall survival rates are 75%, 60%, and 41%, respectively [11]. In several series, nodal stage has been shown to be significantly associated with disease-specific survival.

## Summary

The unknown primary tumor represents several clinical dilemmas including how to find the primary site and, if the site is never found, where to direct treatment. The incidence of patients with an unknown primary site is low overall because of the effectiveness of clinical examination coupled with panendoscopy and directed biopsies. Radiographic technology including CT/MRI, PET scan, and, more recently, PET-CT may be of value in some cases. As these diagnostic methods become more refined, there may eventually be no patients with an unknown primary tumor. Of course, once the primary site is identified, treatment of these patients can become much more specifically directed. The authors hope that in future editions of head and neck cancer texts the unknown primary site will no longer be a featured entry.

## Acknowledgments

The authors thank Osamu Sakai, MD, PhD, and Nirav P. Shah, MD, of the Department of Radiology at Boston Medical Center for images use in this article.

## References

[1] Talmi YP, Wolf GT, Hazuka M, et al. Unknown primary of the head and neck. J Laryngol Otol 1996;110:353–6.
[2] Wang RC, Goepfert H, Barber A. Unknown primary squamous cell carcinoma metastatic to the neck. Arch Otolaryngol Head Neck Surg 1990;116:1388–93.
[3] Mendenhall W, Mancuso A, Parsons J, et al. Diagnostic evaluation of squamous cell carcinoma metastatic to cervical lymph nodes from an unknown head and neck primary site. Head Neck 1998;20:739–44.
[4] DeSanto L, Neel H. Squamous cell carcinoma: metastasis to the neck from an unknown or undiscovered primary. Otolaryngol Clin North Am 1985;18:505–13.
[5] Chepeha D, Koch W, Pitman K. Management of unknown primary tumor. Head Neck 2003; 6:499–504.
[6] Aasar O, Fischbein N, Caputo G, et al. Metastatic head and neck cancer: role and usefulness of FDG PET in locating occult primary tumors. Radiology 1999;210:177–81.
[7] Johansen J, Eigtved A, Buchwald C, et al. Implication of 18F-fluoro-2-deoxy-D-glucose positron emission tomography on management of carcinoma of unknown primary in the head and neck: a Danish cohort study. Laryngoscope 2002;112:2009–14.
[8] Schoder H, Yeung H, Gonen M, et al. Head and neck cancer: clinical usefulness and accuracy of PET/CT image fusion. Radiology 2004;231:65–72.
[9] Mendenhall W, Mancuso A, Amdur R, et al. Squamous cell carcinoma metastatic to the neck from an unknown head and neck primary site. Am J Otolaryngol 2001;22:261–7.
[10] McQuone S, Eisele D, Lee D, et al. Occult tonsillar carcinoma in the unknown primary. Laryngoscope 1998;108:1605–10.
[11] Colletier P, Garden A, Morrison W, et al. Postoperative radiation for squamous cell carcinoma metastatic to cervical lymph nodes from an unknown primary site: outcomes and patterns of failure. Head Neck 1998;20:674–81.

[12] Davidson B, Sprio R, Patel S, et al. Cervical metastases of occult origin: the impact of combined modality therapy. Am J Surg 1994;168:395–9.

[13] Weir L, Keane T, Cummings B, et al. Radiation treatment of cervical lymph node metastases from an unknown primary: an analysis of outcome by treatment volume and other prognostic factors. Radiother Oncol 1995;35:206–11.

[14] Tong C, Luk M, Chow S, et al. Cervical nodal metastases from occult primary: undifferentiated carcinoma versus squamous cell carcinoma. Head Neck 2002;24:361–9.

[15] Harper C, Mendenhall W, Parsons J, et al. Cancer in neck nodes with unknown primary site: role of mucosal radiotherapy. Head Neck 1990;12:463–9.

[16] Carlson L, Fletcher G, Oswald M. Guidelines for radiotherapeutic techniques for cervical metastases from an unknown primary. Int J Radiat Oncol Biol Phys 1986;12:2101–10.

[17] Reddy S, Marks J. Metastatic carcinoma in the cervical lymph nodes from an unknown primary site: results of bilateral neck plus mucosal irradiation vs. ipsilateral neck irradiation. Int J Radiat Oncol Biol Phys 1997;37:797–802.

[18] Fritz M, Esclamado R, Lorenz R, et al. Recurrence rates after selective neck dissection in the N0 irradiated neck. Arch Otolaryngol Head Neck Surg 2002;128:292–5.

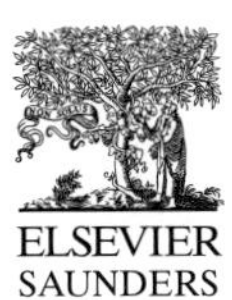ELSEVIER
SAUNDERS

Otolaryngol Clin N Am
38 (2005) 99–105

OTOLARYNGOLOGIC
CLINICS
OF NORTH AMERICA

# Management of the Neck in Salivary Gland Carcinoma

Daniel R. Gold, MD,
Donald J. Annino, Jr, MD, DMD*

*Department of Otolaryngology, Tufts University School of Medicine,
New England Medical Center, 750 Washington Street,
Boston, MA 02111, USA*

Major salivary gland malignancies are rare tumors, representing between 1% and 3% of head and neck cancers and 0.3% of all cancers [1]. This incidence, in conjunction with the variety of histologic types and grades, makes a consensus on the treatment of salivary gland cancers particularly challenging. It is difficult for any single institution to accrue a significant number of patients prospectively in less than a decade. It is also difficult to predict prognosis because of the tendency of these tumors for delayed recurrence. Therefore, there is no single accepted approach to the management of the neck, particularly the N0 neck, in patients with major salivary gland malignancies.

## Treatment of the primary tumor

The treatment of the primary in salivary gland tumors is well accepted and includes, when possible, resection of the primary tumor. As with any cancer resection, the goal is to resect all clinical disease with a curative attempt. This primary resection frequently includes the paraparotid and periparotid lymph nodes, which can provide an important prognostic tool. Postoperative radiation to the primary bed has been proven to be beneficial for tumors with aggressive histology, large size, or facial nerve involvement. Leverstein et al [2] found that among patients with tumors dissected off the facial nerve, postoperative radiation significantly decreased locoregional 5- and 10-year recurrence rates.

* Corresponding author.

*E-mail address:* dannino@tufts-nemc.org (D.J. Annino, Jr).

0030-6665/05/$ - see front matter © 2005 Elsevier Inc. All rights reserved.
doi:10.1016/j.otc.2004.09.006     *oto.theclinics.com*

## Treatment of the neck

The treatment of the neck presents more of a challenge. Although the reported incidence of clinical cervical metastasis is only 16% for parotid gland and 8% for the other major salivary gland malignancies [3], nodal disease has a significant effect on prognosis. Most reports show poorer outcomes in patients with clinical cervical disease than in those without cervical disease. Battacharyya et al [4] demonstrated a 50% decrease in mean survival in patients with neck disease versus those without disease. Shah [5] and Kelley and Spiro [6] corroborate a similar significant decrease in 5-year survival in both parotid and submandibular gland malignancy. The current most widely accepted treatment of the neck in salivary gland malignancy is summarized in Fig. 1.

### The N-positive neck

The approach to clinically positive nodal disease is well accepted and well standardized. Therapeutic neck dissection is the accepted treatment for patients with clinically obvious cervical nodal involvement. The extent of the neck dissection is determined by the grossly involved lymph nodes, and an attempt should be made to spare vital structures. The most common levels of the neck involved are levels II and III [3]. Because contralateral neck involvement is rare, only the ipsilateral neck is usually treated. Many studies have shown that there is improved locoregional control and increased survival with the addition of postoperative radiation. Armstrong et al [7] evaluated patients with salivary malignancy and surgical treatment of clinical neck disease and found a 5-year local control rate of 69% in those

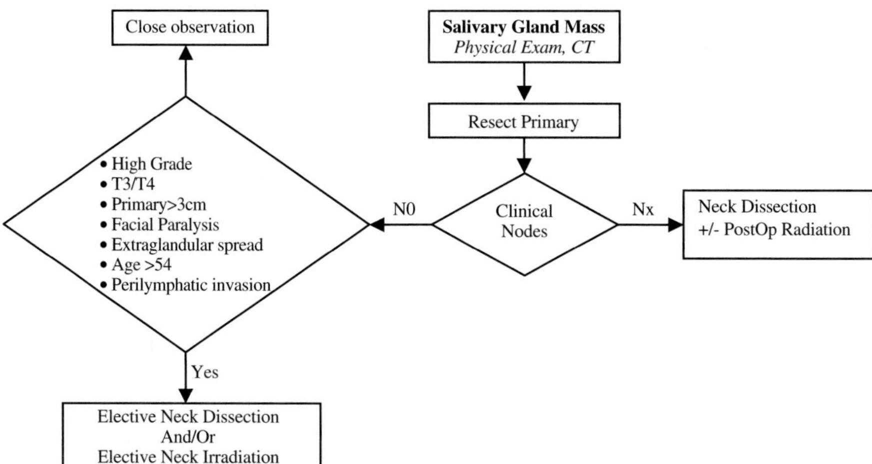


Fig. 1. Summary of treatment of neck in major salivary gland malignancy.

who received postsurgical radiation versus a 40% control rate in those treated with surgery alone. Similarly 5-year survival rates were higher in the group treated with surgery and radiation group (49%) than in the group treated with surgery alone (19%). Therefore, most institutions favor postoperative radiation therapy in patients with clinical neck disease in an attempt to treat any additional occult disease that may exist after dissection.

## The N0 neck

Treatment of the clinically negative neck has been more controversial. The treatment of the N0 neck in major salivary gland malignancies has included observation, elective neck dissection, and primary radiation. Currently, there are differing recommendations in the literature as the best treatment. The reason for treating at all is the hope of eradicating any micrometastatic, occult disease. Because elective neck dissection and radiation therapy seem to have equivalent outcomes, the choice is based on the features of the primary tumor or on patient or clinician preference. Thus, in general, treatment of the N0 neck is appropriate when the risk for occult metastasis is high.

## Predictive factors

The reported incidence of occult lymph node metastasis varies from 12% to 48% [6]. A number of studies have looked at possible predictive factors for the presence of occult metastatic neck disease. The strongest predictors of occult disease have been histology, pathologic grade, stage, and size of the primary lesion [6]. Pain and involvement of the facial nerve have also been found to be predictors of occult metastasis [4,6]. Weaker associations have been shown with age greater than 54 years at diagnosis, extraglandular involvement, and lymphatic invasion [6].

Intuitively, the histology of the primary salivary gland malignancy should be an important factor in the risk of occult metastasis. In fact, during the past decades several studies have shown that certain tumor pathologies carry a powerful significant trend in the risk of occult nodal involvement, and others do not. The incidence is found to be higher in anaplastic, high-grade mucoepidermoid, squamous cell, adenocarcinoma, and salivary duct carcinoma than in low-grade mucoepidermoid and acinic cell carcinoma (Table 1) [1,3,4,8]. In general high-grade tumors are more frequently associated with occult metastasis than are low-grade tumors. One recent study differs slightly from the others. Stenert et al [8] reported higher-than-expected occult nodal disease in the accepted low-risk pathologies. The incidence was still significantly less than for the high-grade tumors but was greater than seen in other reports. The significance if this finding is unclear, because the reported survival in this study is the same as that of the rest of the literature.

Table 1
Risk of occult disease based on histology of primary tumor

| High risk | Low risk |
| --- | --- |
| Squamous cell carcinoma | Adenoid cystic |
| Adenocarcinoma | Acinic cell |
| High-grade Mucoepidermoid | Low-grade mucoepidermoid |
| Undifferentiated malignant mixed salivary duct carcinoma | Sarcoma |
| Expleomorphic adenoma | |

An increased risk of occult disease is also associated with advanced-stage disease. Armstrong et al [3] found that among patients with N0 necks, T4 lesions had a 24% risk of occult cervical disease, versus 16% for T3 lesions and 7% for T1/T2 lesions. They also showed an independent increased risk for primary tumors larger than 3 cm (20%) versus those smaller than 3 cm (4%).

Facial nerve paralysis has long been recognized as a prognostic factor in local recurrence, and recent studies have also shown an association with an increased risk of regional disease. Frankenthaler et al [9] showed that occult nodal metastases were more common in the presence of facial nerve paralysis (80%) than in the absence of facial nerve involvement (19%). Similarly, Califano et al [10] observed facial paralysis in 69% of patients with nodal metastasis but in only 21% of patients without nodal metastasis.

*N0 treatment*

The treatment of the N0 neck in major salivary gland malignancies has included observation, elective neck dissection, and primary radiation. Some of these recommendations have been based on the data obtained from the statistics and treatment of squamous cell carcinoma of the head and neck. Care must be exercised in using these data, because there is no proof in the literature that malignancy of the major salivary glands behaves or responds in a fashion similar to squamous cell carcinoma of mucosal origin. In fact, given the range of histologic types of salivary gland cancers, it is unlikely their treatment and response will be the same as mucosally derived squamous cell carcinoma.

*Surgery*

Historically, observation and possibly radiation of the neck have been the treatment for occult cervical metastasis. There have been reports recommending surgery, in particular recent reports from Europe. If elective neck dissection is to be performed, levels I through III need to be addressed. Armstrong et al [3] have shown that with clinically positive necks a thorough neck dissection is needed. They found metastasis from parotid primary tumors frequently involves level II and level II cervical nodes; however, up to 25% of lesions skipped to levels III and IV. Their findings are slightly different in elective N0 neck dissections. With an N0 neck, they found if levels I through III were removed all occult disease was removed. No occult disease was found in levels IV or V. Bardwil [11] also recommended dissection of first-echelon nodes in all salivary gland malignancies. This limited dissection was believed to add minimal morbidity to the primary resection and to be adequate treatment.

Recently, European centers have recommended elective neck dissection in all patients with major salivary gland malignancies, including N0 necks. Zbaren et al [12] recommend elective neck dissection in all N0 necks, removing levels I through III. They also recommend postoperative radiation therapy in all patients staged T2 through T4. Their survival and recurrence rates are no different from those reported in the literature treated by radiation alone. Their main reason for recommending surgery is that frequently the correct histologic tumor type is not ascertained until after surgery.

Stennart et al [8] recommend elective neck dissection on all major salivary gland malignancies because they believe most salivary gland tumors have poor radiosensitivity and because a similar approach is used in other head and neck cancers. Despite their performing an elective neck dissection on every patient, however, their 5-year survival rate is no different from the literature recommending radiation therapy without a neck dissection.

Johns [13], who advocates treating the neck based on histology and stage of the primary tumor, suggests a more focused surgical treatment plan. He recommends no neck dissection for T1/T2 disease but neck dissection with or without postoperative radiotherapy for all T3/T4 primary tumors. Spiro et al [14] further refine this recommendation to include elective neck dissection for what they consider very high-risk histology (ie, anaplastic or squamous cell carcinoma). Kelly and Spiro [6] include in these indications all high-grade malignancies or any primary tumor larger than 4 cm.

Most authors who recommend surgery for the N0 neck do so to avoid radiation if possible. They prefer to leave radiation as an option in the future. In patients who are found to have occult positive adenopathy after an elective neck dissection, as with the clinically positive neck, surgical dissection and radiation may be used as complementary techniques. Jackson [15] suggests performing an upper neck dissection along with the primary resection. If sampled nodes are positive, the neck should be treated with radiation therapy. On the other hand, if sampled nodes are negative for occult disease, and no other indications for radiation exist, patients may be spared the cost and morbidity of radiation. Kormaz et al [16] recommend sampling of level I and II nodes with intraoperative frozen-section analysis for high-grade primary tumors. A full neck dissection is performed if frozen samples are positive for occult disease, and radiation therapy is added to control occult disease further in high-risk pathology. Armstrong et al [3] have also shown a benefit from the use of postoperative radiation in patients with clinically N0 necks and subsequent occult positive adenopathy.

*Radiation*

Historically, salivary gland malignancies have been thought to have poor radiosensitivity. This assumption was made because radiation therapy alone was not usually successful in controlling salivary gland malignancies. Newer radiotherapy techniques and options have changed this opinion. Several studies show a clear benefit to the use of radiation following surgery [3,7]. In fact several studies show similar outcomes between elective neck dissection and elective neck irradiation. Armstong et al [3] noted that in a high-risk group with N0 necks, postoperative radiation had a low rate of recurrence with long-term outcome similar to elective neck dissection. Therefore in the patient with a N0 neck who will be treated with radiation for the primary tumor, it is sensible to treat the neck and avoid a neck dissection. Frequently, the characteristics of the primary tumor that place the neck at high risk are the same ones that increase the risk for local recurrence. Elective radiation of the neck is also supported by extensive evidence from the treatment of epidermoid head and neck cancer. Care must be taken, however, before applying these data to salivary histologies that look and behave differently from head and neck squamous cell carcinoma [14].

## Summary

In conclusion, salivary malignancies are a rare group of tumors that are still relatively poorly understood. The management of the neck in major salivary gland malignancies, in particular the treatment of the N0 neck, is controversial. It is difficult for any single institution to accrue a significant number of patients. Multiple histopathologic subtypes and behavior patterns further confuse the management of neck disease.

The treatment of the clinically positive neck is fairly well accepted. Therapeutic neck dissection is the accepted treatment, usually with post-operative radiation.

Treatment of the N0 neck remains more controversial. The current approach favors basing the decision on the histology, stage of the primary tumor, facial nerve involvement, and pain. Those predictive factors are considered reasons for surgery or radiation. A growing number of reports recommend elective neck dissections for all major salivary gland malignancies, but this recommendation is far from universally accepted at this time. These studies not show an increased survival or control with elective neck dissection.

## References

[1] Spitz MR, Batsakis JG. Major salivary gland carcinoma: descriptive epidemiology and survival of 498 patients. Arch Otolaryngol 1984;110:45–9.

[2] Leverstein H, Van Der Wal JE, Tiwani RM, et al. Malignant epithelial parotid gland tumors: analysis and results in 65 previously untreated patients. Br J Surg 1998;85(9):1267–72.

[3] Armstrong JG, Harrison LB, Thaler HT, et al. The indications for elective treatment of the neck in cancer of the major salivary glands. Cancer 1992;69:615–9.

[4] Battacharyya N, Fried MP. Nodal metastasis in major salivary gland cancer: predictive factors and effects on survival. Arch Otolaryngol 2002;128:904–8.

[5] Shah J. Management of regional metastasis in salivary and thyroid cancer. In: Larson D, Ballantyne A, Guillamondegui O, editors. Cancer of the neck: evaluation and treatment. New York: Macmillan Publishing Co; 1986. p. 253–8.

[6] Kelley DJ, Spiro RH. Management of the neck in parotid carcinoma. Am J Surg 1996;172: 695–7.

[7] Armstrong JG, Harrison LB, Spiro RH, et al. Malignant tumors of major salivary gland origin. A matched pair analysis of the role of combined surgery and postoperative radiotherapy. Arch Otolaryngol 1990;116:290–3.

[8] Stennert E, Kisner D, Jungehuelsing M, et al. High incidence of lymph node metastasis in major salivary gland cancer. Arch Otolaryngol 2003;129:720–3.

[9] Frankenthaler RA, Byers RM, Luna MA. Predicting occult lymph nodes metastasis in parotid cancer. Arch Otolaryngol 1993;119:517–20.

[10] Califano L, Zupi A, Massari S, et al. Indication for neck dissection in carcinoma of the parotid gland. International Journal of Surgery 1993;78:347–9.

[11] Bardwil J. Tumors of the parotid gland. Am J Surg 1967;114:498–502.

[12] Zbaren P, Schupbach J, Nuyens M, et al. Carcinoma of the parotid gland. Am J Surg 2003; 186:57–62.

[13] Johns M. Parotid cancer: a rational basis for treatment. Head Neck 1980;3:132–44.

[14] Spiro RH, Armstrong JG, Harrison LB, et al. Carcinoma of major salivary glands. Recent trends. Arch Otolaryngol 1989;115:316–21.

[15] Jackson GL. Management of the neck in parotid cancer [comment]. Am J Surg 1999;177(3): 278.

[16] Kormaz H, Yoo GH, Du W, et al. Predictors of nodal metastasis in salivary gland cancer. J Surg Oncol 2002;80:186–9.

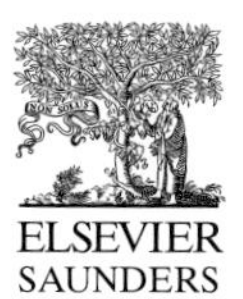

Otolaryngol Clin N Am
38 (2005) 107–131



# Anterior Skull Base Surgery

Michael J. Kaplan, MD[a,b], Nancy J. Fischbein, MD[a,c,*],
Griffith R. Harsh, MD[b]

[a]*Department of Otolaryngology-Head and Neck Surgery, Stanford
University Medical Center, Stanford, CA, USA*
[b]*Department of Neurological Surgery, Stanford University
Medical Center, Stanford, CA, USA*
[c]*Division of Neuroradiology, Stanford University
Medical Center, Stanford, CA, USA*

The goals of anterior skull base surgery have remained constant throughout the continuing evolution of surgical and radiation oncology techniques. These goals include

1. Resection of tumor with negative margins
2. Preservation of neurologic function, including vision and olfaction
3. Reduction of operative complications through
   a. Minimal brain retraction
   b. Segregation of intracranial contents from the contaminated paranasal sinuses
4. Improved aesthetic outcome

Surgical approaches to the anterior skull base have evolved since an initial paper in 1954 by Smith [1] described resection of a frontal sinus tumor. Before Smith's report, two papers appeared in which an orbital tumor had been resected through a craniotomy [2] or a craniotomy-transorbital approach [3]. Between 1963 and 1973, Ketcham et al [4] and Van Buren et al [5] demonstrated clearly that surgery in this area improves the likelihood of cure for malignancies, even with the significant associated morbidity. Since that time, numerous surgical techniques have been introduced to extend or improve anatomic access for resection or reconstruction or to reduce functional or aesthetic morbidity. Small transfacial incisions that supplement a bicoronal craniotomy incision are widely used [6], and, increasingly, endoscopic and endoscopic-assisted

* Corresponding author. 300 Pasteur Drive, Stanford, CA 94305.
*E-mail address:* fischbein@stanford.edu (N.J. Fischbein).

0030-6665/05/$ - see front matter © 2005 Elsevier Inc. All rights reserved.
doi:10.1016/j.otc.2004.09.010

approaches are being perfected for selected cases, as reviewed by Har-El [7]. Today, anterior skull base surgery by experienced multidisciplinary teams is internationally performed and accepted, with documented improved local control and survival compared with a generation ago and with severe morbidity and mortality reduced to less than 5% [8].

This review focuses on selected key anatomic considerations, briefly reviews common pathologies of the paranasal sinuses, and provides an overview of surgical approaches, complications, and results.

## Surgical anatomy

The anterior skull base includes the posterior frontal sinus, cribriform plate, and roof of the orbit and ethmoid sinus. More posteriorly, it includes the planum sphenoidale, anterior aspect of the roof of the sphenoid sinus, and lesser wing of the sphenoid bone. Details of this anatomy are well reviewed by Lang [8a] and, from an endoscopic point of view, by Jho and Ha [9]. A number of aspects of this anatomy are particularly pertinent to the surgeon.

### Orbit preservation

Some controversy remains regarding how much of the orbit can be involved by tumor and still have its functional integrity preserved at surgery. Some believe that involvement of the lamina papyracea demands orbital exenteration. Many others, including the authors, believe that the orbit can be functionally preserved in an oncologically sound fashion if there is no significant involvement of the orbital fat, even if the orbital periosteum is involved. The thin fascial layer that surrounds the orbital fat just inside the orbital periosteum probably accounts for the ability to resect significant periosteum and still maintain orbital integrity [10] (Fig. 1). In the authors' experience, when the patient has full extraocular motility on clinical examination, one can usually preserve the orbit. If there is diplopia solely because of mass effect leading to proptosis and interference with extraocular muscle function but without radiologically evident orbital fat extension, the orbit can probably be preserved. Although MRI is extremely helpful in evaluating the orbit, the final decision with regard to orbit preservation may have to be made intraoperatively (Fig. 2).

### Preservation of vision; protection internal carotid artery

The ophthalmic artery arises from the internal carotid artery (ICA) superiorly or superomedially and then courses through the optic canal along the optic nerve. It typically runs on the lateral surface of the nerve at the anterior optic canal. Thus, dissection of the anterior optic chiasm and the medial optic canal is generally safe.

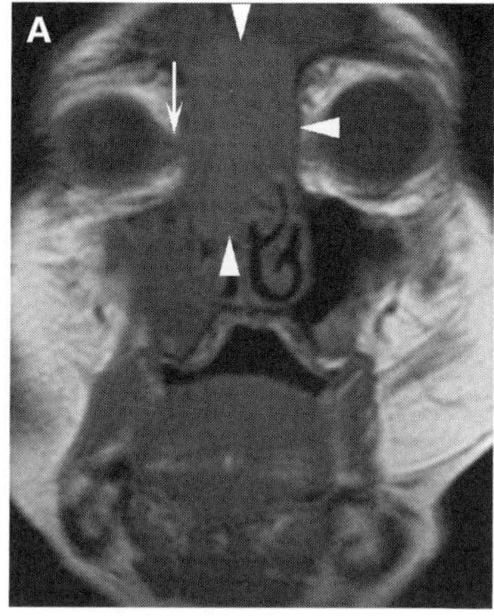
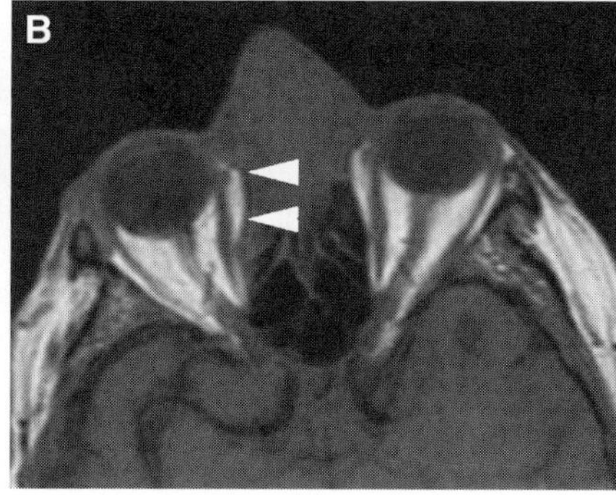

Fig. 1. An 80-year-old woman with a history of poorly differentiated SCC of the frontal and ethmoid sinuses also involving the nasal cavity and extending to skin and previously treated with radiation presenting with recurrent disease. (*A*) A coronal T1-weighted image demonstrates a large soft tissue mass filling the nasal cavity and ethmoid sinuses, extending superiorly into the frontal sinuses (*arrowheads*). Although tumor approaches the medial canthal region (*arrow*), the orbital fat is uninvolved. (*B*) An axial T1-weighted image demonstrates the intact right lamina papyracea (*arrowheads*) and the uninvolved orbital fat. A subfrontal craniectomy approach was used for resection, with radial free flap reconstruction. A neck dissection was also performed. The orbit was preserved, and no medial canthal ligament reconstruction was necessary. No diplopia was present postoperatively.

The optic nerve and ICA are usually covered by bone in the superolateral aspect of the sphenoid sinus, although in some cases the bone may be dehiscent. The optic nerve lies just superior to the ICA.

Careful review of the preoperative MRI is essential to understand the anatomic relationships in a particular patient. In some cases, an intraoperative navigation system is useful to guide resection near vital structures, and a preoperative MRI scan is required for intraoperative navigation purposes.

## Cribriform plate and dura

The olfactory apparatus lies just above the cribriform plate, which itself lies just medial and usually slightly inferior to the ethmoid roof. Dura is much more tightly adherent at the cribriform plate than at the ethmoid roof. A thin-section (1 mm) coronal CT scan is useful for assessing the bony integrity of the cribriform plate and ethmoid roof. This area can also be assessed with MRI, which better depicts dural and parenchymal extension of tumor. Thin-section coronal fast spin echo T2-weighted images are often most useful for assessing the presence or absence of subtle anterior skull base penetration, whereas coronal postgadolinium T1-weighted images with fat saturation most sensitively demonstrate or exclude dural, leptomeningeal,

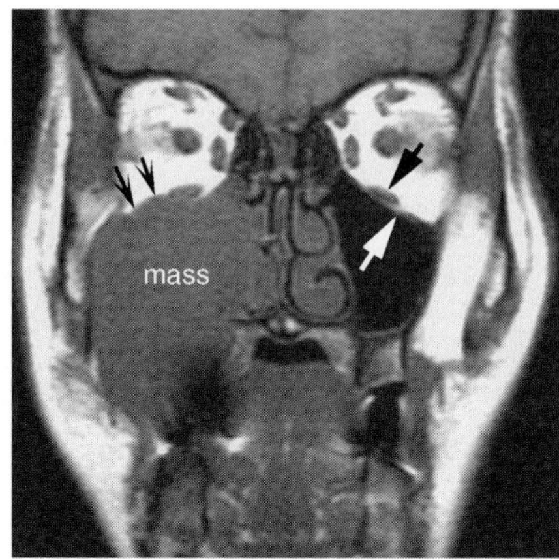


Fig. 2. A 35-year-old woman with adenocarcinoma of the maxillary sinus demonstrating minimal restriction of upward gaze and decreased sensation in the V2 distribution on clinical examination. A coronal T1-weighted image demonstrates a large mass centered on the right maxillary sinus, with tumor extending into the inferior aspect of the right orbit (*black concave arrows*). The normal left inferior rectus (*black straight arrow*) and normal infraorbital nerve (*white arrow*) are indicated. From the image, although there is clearly intraorbital extension of tumor, it is not possible to say whether orbital periosteum is invaded or breached. At surgery, the orbital periosteum and V2 were removed, but orbital fat and inferior rectus muscle were uninvolved, and the orbit was spared. The patient received postoperative IMRT to a dose of 70 Gy, and she has no evidence of disease at 4-year follow-up.

and parenchymal extension (Fig. 3). If the olfactory apparatus is involved only minimally and unilaterally, one can consider whether preservation of the contralateral olfactory apparatus is feasible. For example, possible preservation is an issue in the resection of selected small esthesioneuroblastomas. If preserving the contralateral system results in inadequate exposure for complete tumor resection using the craniotomy approach, an external ethmoidectomy or endoscopic supplementation is required.

*Limits of resectability*

Poor clinical prognostic indicators include dural and especially brain involvement. Orbital involvement and extension of tumor to the pterygoid plates, infratemporal fossa, or nasopharynx are also indicators of poor prognosis (Fig. 4). Although involvement of these areas portends a worse prognosis, it is not an absolute contraindication for surgery, and proceeding with surgery may be worthwhile. For example, Fee et al [11], Ibrahim et al [12], and To et al [13,14] have demonstrated that resection of the soft tissue and cartilage of the nasopharynx can be done effectively in selected cases of recurrent nasopharyngeal carcinoma. The authors and others have resected tumors that extend to the infratemporal fossa and greater wing of the sphenoid with acceptable morbidity and with long-term results dependent largely on the underlying histology. Malignant tumors that extend to the

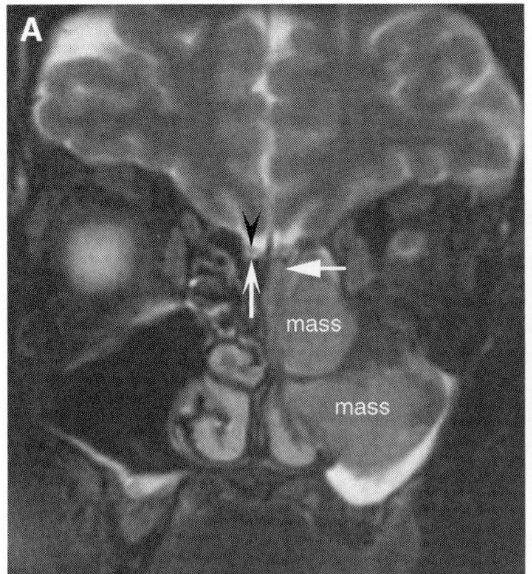

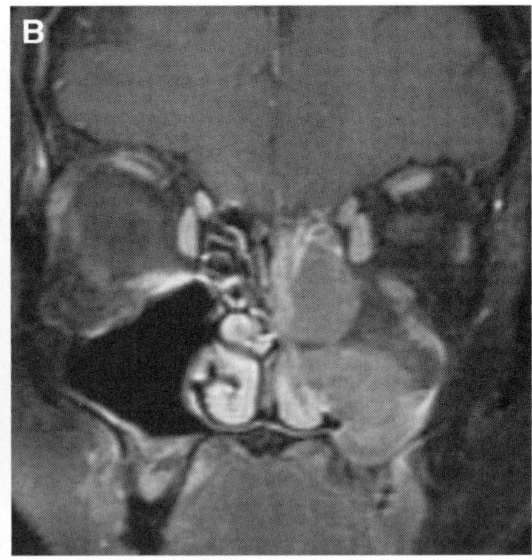


Fig. 3. A 55-year-old woman with SCC of the maxillary and ethmoid sinuses and with involvement of the nasal cavity presented for preoperative evaluation. (*A*) Coronal fast spin echo T2-weighted image with fat saturation demonstrates a lobulated mass in the left maxillary and ethmoid sinuses, as well as tumor extending superiorly in the olfactory recess (*straight white arrow*) toward the anterior cranial fossa. The normal right cribriform plate (*concave white arrow*) and right olfactory bulb (*concave black arrowhead*) are shown. Although tumor seems to abut the left cribriform plate, the left olfactory apparatus is well seen, and there is no evidence of tumor penetration of the anterior cranial fossa. The orbit is also intact. (*B*) A coronal postgadolinium T1-weighted image with fat saturation shows no abnormal enhancement of dura. These findings were confirmed intraoperatively; the orbit was uninvolved, and the cribriform plate and ethmoid roof were intact. The tumor was resected using a transethmoidal external approach, and the patient received postoperative radiation therapy.

cavernous sinus or the petrous carotid artery, however, are usually regarded as unresectable. Most surgeons also feel that involvement of the optic chiasm is an absolute contraindication for surgery, because the surgery would result in immediate bilateral blindness.

## Preoperative clinical and radiologic assessment

Before a surgical approach to a tumor of the anterior skull base is planned, it is important to exclude histologies for which surgical resection may not be indicated. Establishing that a mass is a metastasis rather than a primary tumor of the anterior skull base should lead to further metastatic evaluation. If additional metastases are found, a palliative approach with chemotherapy may be a better next intervention than skull base surgery. Primary lymphomas of the skull base and paranasal sinuses are common enough to be considered in the differential diagnosis of many aggressive lesions of the anterior skull base (Fig. 5). Biopsy, under CT guidance if necessary, is usually indicated to exclude this condition. On the other hand, there are times that surgical resection might be indicated even for

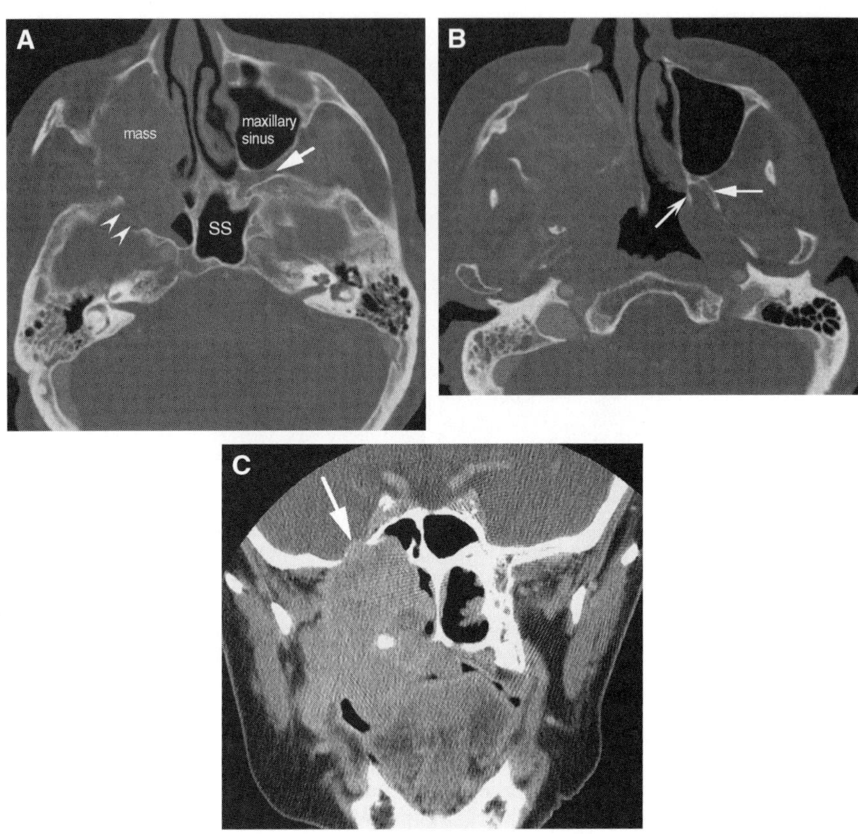

Fig. 4. A 75-year-old woman with a large adenocarcinoma of the maxilla presented for evaluation. (*A*) An axial CT scan in bone window demonstrates a large mass centered on the right maxillary sinus, with extension posteriorly into the pterygopalatine fossa and the sphenoid sinus. The normal left maxillary sinus, pterygopalatine fossa (*white arrow*) and sphenoid sinus (SS) are shown for comparison. In addition, there is focal erosion of the greater wing of the sphenoid on the right (*arrowheads*). (*B*) A more inferior axial CT image in bone window demonstrates complete destruction of the pterygoid plates on the right. The normal left medial (*concave arrow*) and lateral (*straight arrow*) pterygoid plates are shown for comparison. (*C*) A coronal postcontrast CT scan in soft tissue window demonstrates the large mass. The focal defect in the greater wing of the sphenoid is demonstrated, with enhancing tumor extending into the inferomedial aspect of the right middle cranial fossa (*arrow*). The tumor is sharply circumscribed, suggesting that it is extradural or possibly involves dura but does not extend through the dura to invade brain. At surgery the dura was found to be uninvolved. A complete tumor resection with close margins was possible, including involved soft tissue and bone. Postoperative IMRT was given.

a metastasis to the skull base or for an anterior skull base primary tumor with distant metastases. Such surgery with noncurative intent might be undertaken to repair a cerebrospinal fluid (CSF) leak, or if nonsurgical intervention is likely to lead to a CSF leak or a high risk of meningitis. When a surgical procedure is indicated by clinical and imaging findings

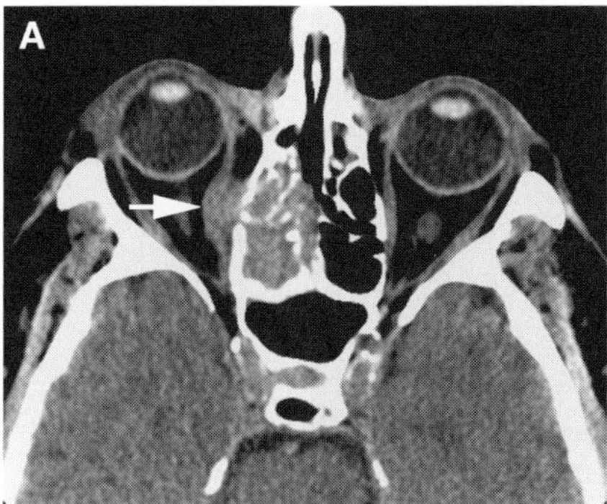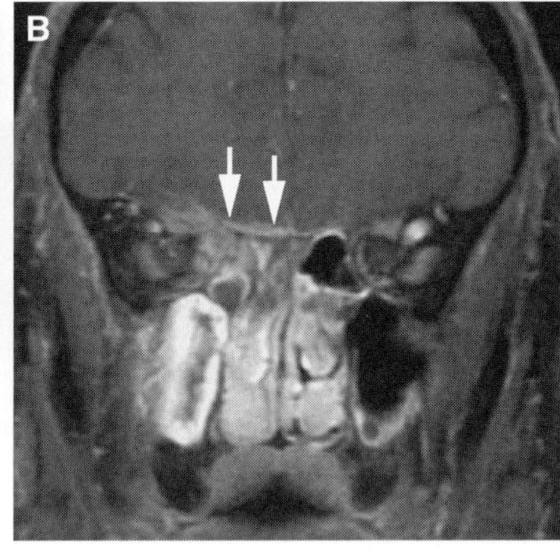

Fig. 5. A 70-year-old man with a history of prior endoscopic sinus surgery presented with right periorbital swelling, mild proptosis, and diplopia. (*A*) An axial noncontrast CT scan in soft tissue window demonstrates soft tissue in the right ethmoid sinus with extension of the process laterally into the right orbit. The medial rectus muscle (*white arrow*) is deviated laterally. (*B*) A coronal postgadolinium T1-weighted image with fat saturation demonstrates intracranial extension of this infiltrative lesion, with irregular thickening and enhancement of the dura (*arrows*). Because lymphoma was a strong consideration in the differential diagnosis, a biopsy was obtained. Biopsy confirmed the diagnosis of non-Hodgkin's lymphoma, and the patient was subsequently evaluated and treated nonsurgically.

whatever the histology, it may be advisable to simply obtain a frozen section at the beginning of the surgical procedure. In a few cases, notably the juvenile angiofibromas, the history, clinical findings, and radiologic findings are pathognomonic, and a biopsy is unnecessary; the histology will be confirmed as part of the definitive resection.

Radiologic imaging facilitates both preoperative planning and subsequent clinical follow-up. A high-quality MRI is usually the initial examination of choice and is sometimes supplemented with coronal CT for assessment of the cribriform plate. In addition to providing the surgeon with critical information regarding the extent of tumor and relationships to important nerves and arteries, the MRI allows assessment of potential perineural spread of tumor along branches of the trigeminal nerve (Fig. 6). In some cases the MRI suggests specific histologies such as primary lymphoma or angiofibroma (Fig. 7). For many histologies, a baseline assessment of the neck is helpful for current treatment planning and future tumor surveillance. Furthermore, if a tumor appears highly vascular, preoperative angiography and embolization should be considered, depending on whether the internal maxillary artery is likely to be a major contributor to the tumor's blood supply. If the tumor's blood supply is likely to be from the anterior and posterior ethmoidal arteries, which are branches of the ophthalmic artery, then these vessels cannot be safely embolized unless vision has already been lost.

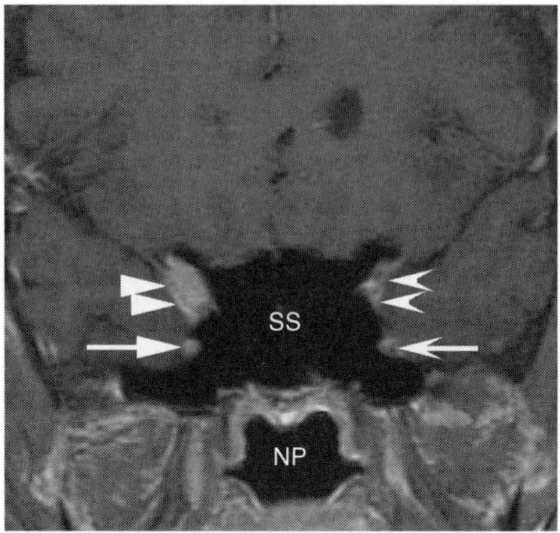

Fig. 6. A 66-year-old man presented for evaluation of SCC of the skin of the forehead with extension into the nasal cavity, ethmoid sinus, and frontal sinus. On examination he was found to be numb over his right forehead and cheek, and a preoperative MRI scan was obtained. A coronal postgadolinium T1-weighted image with fat saturation demonstrated abnormal enhancing soft tissue in the right superior orbital fissure (*straight arrowheads*), consistent with perineural extension of tumor along V1, as well as enlargement and enhancement of V2 (*straight arrow*) secondary to perineural spread of tumor. The normal left superior orbital fissure (*concave arrowheads*) and left V2 in foramen rotundum (*concave arrow*) are shown for comparison. *Abbreviations:* SS, sphenoid sinus; NP, nasopharynx.

Intraoperative navigation, usually with MR-based systems but at times with CT instead, is often helpful to the surgeon, depending on the surgical approach planned and whether the tumor involves important surgical landmarks so that the surgeon's intraoperative localization abilities are compromised. Navigation is also important if the tumor is to be approached using an approach with a narrow vista (such as endoscopic approaches) or when critical structures will be immediately distal to tumor or to an eroded landmark. Dissection near the ICA and optic chiasm, for instance, is often aided by intraoperative navigation.

If positron emission tomography (PET) imaging is to be considered in long-term surveillance, it may be helpful to obtain a preoperative PET scan so that any areas that demonstrate unexpected increased activity can be evaluated. A PET scan should also be considered if unexpected metastases would lead to a reassessment of the indications for surgery. In other words, if surgery with curative intent is futile, then do the potential palliative benefits of surgery still outweigh its risks, or should the patient by managed with nonsurgical palliative methods?

## Selected pathologies

Tumors that may require anterior skull base resection include selected malignant tumors of the paranasal sinuses that extend superiorly through the cribriform plate, ethmoid roof, and planum sphenoidale or posteriorly

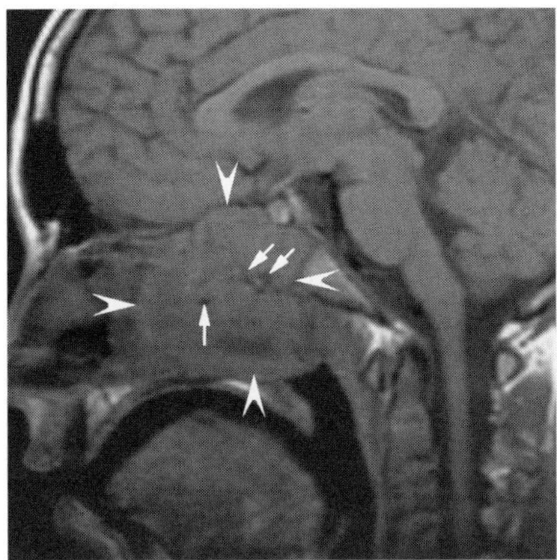

Fig. 7. A 12-year-old boy presented with epistaxis and nasal congestion. A sagittal T1-weighted image demonstrated a large soft tissue mass (*concave arrowheads*) centered in the posterior nasal cavity but extending superiorly into the sphenoid sinus and posteriorly into the nasopharynx. Rounded and serpiginous hypointense structures within the lesion (*small arrows*) are consistent with flow voids. Following preoperative embolization, the lesion was resected, and juvenile angiofibroma was confirmed.

through the posterior wall of the frontal sinus; benign and malignant meningiomas that involve the same area; and selected benign processes such as orbital apex schwannomas, occasional encephaloceles and mucoceles, and selected large benign tumors including juvenile angiofibromas and inverted papillomas. Below are brief overviews of selected histologies [15,16].

### Squamous cell carcinoma

The most common malignancy of the paranasal sinuses is squamous cell carcinoma (SCC). SCC most commonly arises in the maxillary sinus, but extension posteriorly and superomedially may make it necessary to include a skull base resection in overall management. Assessment of the neck is essential in these patients, because approximately 10% of patients present with cervical nodal metastases, and another 20% develop cervical nodal metastases if no elective neck irradiation is included in the treatment plan [17,18]. It is helpful to assess the course of V2 by high-quality, thin-section MRI to evaluate for perineural spread. When indicated for management of skull base extension, skull base surgery with postoperative irradiation has improved the overall local control and cure rates from less than 50% to approximately 60%.

### Adenocarcinoma

Adenocarcinomas account for 10% to 15% of paranasal sinus malignancies in the United States and as many as 40% in Europe, where woodworking and the leather industry are etiologic factors. Surgery plus postoperative irradiation yields local control and cure rates of 45% to 85%. Distant metastases are unusual.

## Adenoid cystic carcinoma

Accounting for 10% to 15% of paranasal sinus malignancies, adenoid cystic carcinoma has a high rate of local recurrence even after appropriate surgery and irradiation. In addition, about 15% to 20% of patients develop hematogenous metastases, usually to the lungs [19]. Because resection of isolated lung metastases is recommended, metastatic evaluations at an appropriate interval are an important component of posttreatment tumor surveillance. Many physicians advise a baseline chest CT scan followed by a periodic chest CT scan every 12 to 18 months. The 5-year local control rate is about 60%, but an additional 15% to 20% of patients with local recurrence can live with disease for significant periods. Although there are few complete responses to chemotherapy, cisplatin-based regimens do seem to be useful for management of recurrent disease. As in SCC, perineural spread is common and should be investigated by high-quality thin-section MRI, both initially and in subsequent surveillance examinations, because there is evidence that radiosurgery along the trigeminal nerve branches and to Meckel's cave and the cavernous sinus is effective in reducing pain and in controlling disease progression.

## Esthesioneuroblastoma (olfactory neuroblastoma)

Esthesioneuroblastomas are rare tumors that arise from the olfactory epithelium and hence are typically seen at the level of the cribriform plate [20–22]. Dural involvement at the level of the olfactory groove is usually present, even when preoperative MRI indicates no apparent involvement superior to the cribriform plate. This involvement makes an anterior skull base approach necessary for management of almost all esthesioneuroblastomas, with the exception of those rare tumors that originate inferior to the olfactory recesses. Extensive involvement of dura and even brain invasion may be present initially or may occur in the context of recurrent disease. Nodal or distant metastases are rare at presentation, but neck metastases develop later in 10% of patients. Several staging classifications have been suggested based either on anatomic extent of disease or assessment of histologic parameters. Histologically aggressive tumors and those that extend to the orbit or dura have a poorer prognosis. In most centers, surgery and radiation therapy are the mainstays of treatment; reported 5-year cure rates are in the range of 61% to 94%. The role of cisplatin-based chemotherapy remains unclear. Some centers routinely use it when there is bone erosion superiorly through the cribriform plate, but others add it for only the most advanced tumors. In addition, there are reports of initial good results using chemotherapy and radiation therapy alone, although follow-up has been short. In most centers, intensity-modulated radiation therapy (IMRT) is preferred. The use of proton beam irradiation has been reported.

## Mucosal melanoma

Melanomas of the nasal cavity and paranasal sinuses are associated with a poor prognosis because of high rates of local recurrence and of distant metastases [23,24]. Surgery and postoperative irradiation are commonly employed. Protocols involving interferon and chemotherapy are available. The 5-year survival rate has been reported to be in the range of 14% to 47%, with most reports in the range of 20% to 25%. When recurrences can be surgically resected with a minimum of morbidity, this resection may be indicated to help maintain a nasal airway and reduce epistaxis.

## Sinonasal undifferentiated carcinoma

Sinonasal undifferentiated carcinoma is a rare, highly aggressive malignancy that commonly presents with extensive local involvement and often involves the orbit and skull base [25,26]. Neck metastases are seen in 20% of patients at presentation. Multimodality therapy is generally used, although there is no consensus on specific irradiation fractionation or chemotherapy protocols. The possibility that these tumors are of neuroendocrine origin has prompted use of cisplatin and etoposide (VP-16) in some regimens. Aggressive surgery, chemotherapy, and IMRT have resulted in longer disease-free intervals than in the past, but prognosis remains poor. Use of proton beam radiotherapy in conjunction with cisplatin and VP-16, often with surgery, has been reported in 13 patients to yield a 3-year overall survival rate of 59% [27]. The goals of treatment are to control local disease, to preserve vision, and to limit significant intracranial extension.

## Chordoma

Approximately one third of chordomas arise in the clivus and extend toward the craniocervical junction. Another 15% occur in cervical vertebrae, and the remainder are sacrococcygeal in origin. The typical age at presentation is 35 to 50 years. Typical symptoms are headache and diplopia secondary to cranial nerve VI paresis; sensory V deficits are common. The extent of other cranial nerve deficits depends on the extent and location of the tumor. Chordomas are often large at presentation and may abut or encase the cavernous segment of the ICA or the vertebrobasilar system. MRI demonstrates a typical imaging appearance in most cases, with a midline location, very high signal intensity on T2-weighted images, and heterogeneous gadolinium enhancement. MRI is useful in assessing the extent of disease and planning surgical approach. Treatment is as complete a resection as possible by an appropriate approach, followed by particle irradiation.

Although the MRI appearance is characteristic enough that the diagnosis can be strongly suspected preoperatively, frozen-section confirmation at the beginning of a resection is advised. Pathology typically shows physaliphorous cells with abundant mucous or glycogen-rich vacuoles, mucoid microcysts, and fibrovascular strands and cords of eosinophilic syncytial cells. Results of surgery plus charged-particle irradiation have shown a 76% to 80% 5-year survival for previously untreated tumors smaller than 75 cm$^3$. About 90% of tumors at the skull base fall into this favorable category. Larger or recurrent tumors do less well, with a 5-year cure rate of about 33%.

*Lymphoma*

Lymphomas represent about 10% of nonepithelial malignancies of the paranasal sinuses. Diffuse large cell B-cell lymphoma is most common, usually presenting as stage 1E. With current multimodality therapy, two thirds of these patients are cured. CD56(+) NK/T-cell lymphomas, usually also Epstein-Barr virus–positive, represent about a third of lymphomas when predominantly nasal involvement is seen. Although some studies from Asia suggest a poorer prognosis, most patients survive. If a lymph node for fine-needle aspiration or biopsy is unavailable, or if the lymph node fine-needle aspiration is insufficient for diagnosis, nasal biopsy is necessary to establish the diagnosis.

*Angiofibroma*

Juvenile angiofibromas are locally expansile, highly vascular benign tumors that occur in male adolescents. Common symptoms are epistaxis and nasal obstruction. Originating at the junction of the posterolateral nasal wall and sphenoid rostrum near the sphenopalatine foramen, they frequently extend laterally into the pterygopalatine fossa, superoposteriorly into the sphenoid sinus, or superiorly to involve the skull base. Anterior extension results in nasal obstruction. The appearance on MRI of a tumor with macroscopic flow voids at this location in an adolescent male is rarely confused with another diagnosis. Juvenile angiofibromas are best resected after preoperative embolization of the tumor and of the ipsilateral internal maxillary artery. Surgical approaches may include a trans-sphenoethmoid approach, a transpalatal approach, or a maxillotomy approach, depending on the extent of tumor and the surgeon's preference. If the tumor extends to the greater wing of the sphenoid, a preauricular orbito-zygomatic approach (sometimes coupled with a middle cranial fossa approach) may be necessary.

**Surgical approaches**

At each institution where skull base surgery is done, the experience of the individual surgeons shapes the decision as to which approach is most appropriate for a particular tumor in a particular patient. This judgment is influenced by the known or suspected histology and whether there has been prior irradiation or surgical intervention, as well as by the patient's preferences regarding risks and alternatives. Key anatomic issues that affect this decision include adequate access for tumor resection with negative margins, the angle of approach so as to minimize brain retraction, the extent of dural or intradural extension, and the need for access to difficult sites such as the optic chiasm, lateral sphenoid sinus recess, nasopharynx, lesser wing of the sphenoid, or craniocervical junction. Anatomically circumscribing the tumor in three dimensions before its actual excision usually affords the best chance of complete resection with frozen-section control of margins. At times, some piecemeal endoscopic resection is strategically planned as part of the resection.

*Bifrontal craniotomy approach with limited transfacial incision*

The anterior skull base has classically been approached through a bifrontal craniotomy with elevation of the frontal lobe or lobes, combined with a transfacial approach to supplement the paranasal sinus exposure. A limited external ethmoidectomy incision that extends inferiorly along the nose to the axial plane of the inferior nasal bone provides adequate exposure for most procedures. There is rarely a need for a lateral rhinotomy or a Weber-Ferguson approach that splits the upper lip. If the hard palate requires extirpation, then an intraoral supplementary approach is added. This combined craniotomy and trans-sphenoethmoid approach provides excellent exposure from the optic chiasm to the spheno-occipital junction, including the planum sphenoidale, orbital roof, frontal sinuses, ethmoid sinuses, sphenoid sinus, and nasopharynx. The medial, superior, and inferior orbit is well exposed, as are the maxilla and nose. The trans-sphenoethmoid component also provides access to the pterygomaxillary fissure and pterygopalatine fossa, pterygoid plate, and nasopharynx. Preoperative MRI, supplemented at times by CT, affords the surgeon a full anatomic map of the tumor and delineates its proximity to critical anatomy.

Intraoperative magnification, microscopic dissection, modern high-speed drills, and, when needed, preoperative tumor embolization have significantly improved operative capability. Repair of CSF leakage and segregation of the brain from the paranasal sinuses is afforded by a pericranial or pericranial-galeal flap, which is usually readily available.

The major advantage of this approach is superb exposure and its familiarity to most skull base surgeons, because it incorporates the key features of a common surgical external ethmoidectomy approach to the paranasal sinuses. It also allows access to uninvolved orbital periosteum either anteriorly or inferiorly, allowing development of a plane between tumor and involved periosteum if orbital preservation is planned.

This approach does have two potentially significant disadvantages: retraction of at least one frontal lobe, and, except in the case of carefully selected anterior tumors, loss of the sense of smell. Brain retraction can be minimized with CSF drainage, usually by a lumbar subarachnoid drain. For tumors extending posteriorly along the planum sphenoidale, temporary removal of the orbital roof affords an angle of exposure that reduces the need for frontal lobe retraction.

### Bifrontal craniotomy approach without supplemental skin or mucosal incisions

With experience and at times with endoscopic assistance from below, surgeons have learned that paranasal exposure is often adequate without a supplemental facial incision [28]. Endoscopes can be used either to guide incisions from above at margins or to guide transnasal planned piecemeal excision of tumor from below [29–31]. Endoscopic-assisted approaches have been used for selected angiofibromas [32,33] and for other tumors and to access the lateral recess of the sphenoid sinus [34].

### Subcranial approach

Raveh et al [35] have popularized the subcranial approach through a bicoronal incision that was initially described for trauma but has been extended to tumor resection. The major advantage of this low craniotomy is minimization of brain retraction, similar to adding a temporary removal of the orbital rim to the classic bifrontal craniotomy. A potential disadvantage of the subcranial approach when it is used in resection of malignant tumors is osteomyelitis or osteoradionecrosis of the disconnected and replaced bone that includes the medial orbital rim, glabella, and part of the nasal bone. The aesthetic deformity that results from removal of this osteomyelitic bone or osteoradionecrotic bone is greater than with a more superior craniotomy. If this region of bone is involved by tumor so that its resection is required, the subcranial approach is ideal. Repair of the dura is similar to that in a bifrontal craniotomy.

### Supplemental midfacial degloving intraoral incision (with or without LeFort I osteotomy or maxillotomy)

A midfacial degloving approach is a well-recognized approach to the paranasal sinuses that avoids a facial incision. It can supplement either a bifrontal craniotomy or a subcranial approach. Some surgeons find this approach helpful, and some patients are strongly adverse to any facial scar, even the small and well-camouflaged one that results from an external ethmoidectomy. Its advantages and disadvantages with respect to angle of exposure and potential complications have been well delineated in the literature. A LeFort I osteotomy may be added, especially if approaching the craniocervical junction. A unilateral maxillotomy approach that mobilizes the inferior maxilla while keeping it attached to the soft palate can also be used [36]. Some find this technique useful if access to the central skull base is needed.

*Endoscopic approach without craniotomy*

Highly selected tumors of the anterior skull base have been resected solely through an endoscopic approach by highly experienced endoscopic surgeons. Described for esthesioneuroblastoma [37], such an approach takes advantage of intraoperative image-guided navigation, specialized equipment, acquired surgical skill, and acceptance of the fact that CSF leaks can be effectively managed by endoscopic repair using autologous sources such as bovine pericardium or other material. After endoscopic total ethmoidectomy and medial maxillectomy are performed as needed, a frontal sinusotomy is done to expose the posterior wall of the frontal sinus lateral to the tumor on each side, and the anterior cranial fossa is then approached extradurally or intradurally through this wall. Dissection continues posteriorly as far as needed; even the optic chiasm can be approached by this method.

*Orbito-zygomatic approach*

Access to the superior parapharyngeal space as well as access along the floor of the middle cranial fossa can be gained by a temporary en bloc removal of the zygomatic arch, lateral orbit, and part of the zygomatic body. This approach may at times be needed to supplement an anterior cranial base approach to provide superolateral access to the foramen ovale, posterolateral maxillary antrum, pterygomaxillary space, lateral orbit, greater wing of the sphenoid, and floor of the middle cranial fossa.

**Areas of controversy**

With the low incidence of anterior skull base tumors, it is difficult to accrue patients for randomized, controlled studies of various therapeutic approaches. Hence, there remain aspects of surgical management that are handled differently by individual surgeons based on their own and their institutional experience. Some of these areas are discussed briefly.

*Can the contralateral sense of smell be preserved when an esthesioneuroblastoma seems to involve only the ipsilateral olfactory bulb at the cribriform plate?*

Preserving the contralateral sense of smell is difficult and should be considered only in highly selected patients. Good-quality thin-section coronal MR images are very helpful in determining whether the opposite CN1 can be spared. The issues are that the opposite CN1 is quite fragile and may be damaged in any case, and the space to repair the CSF leak becomes narrow when one preserves the crista galli. The surgical margin is also closer in these cases. Given the relatively good response to the combination of surgery and postoperative irradiation, and given that there are some who advocate nonsurgical treatment involving only radiation and chemotherapy, some patients might opt to accept a closer surgical margin rather than necessarily sacrifice smell. In highly selected patients, the authors have occasionally successfully preserved the opposite CN1 while obtaining both clean surgical margins and an effective CSF leak repair using a pericranial flap. The approach used has been a bifrontal craniotomy but with dissection at the skull base limited to the affected side, supplemented if needed with either an endoscopic-assisted approach or a small external ethmoidectomy incision.

*Orbit preservation: how much of the medial orbit can be involved and still achieve both an oncologically sound resection and useful eye function?*

The controversial topic of orbit conservation was discussed earlier in this article. Some believe that involvement of the lamina papyracea is an indication for orbit exenteration. More authorities believe that bone involvement per se does not require exenteration, but orbital periosteal involvement does. One can, however, remove considerable periosteum and still maintain conjugate vision without diplopia if the medial and lateral canthal ligaments are preserved and no involvement of orbital fat is found intraoperatively. MRI is helpful in assessing the orbit, but one cannot always definitely establish the presence or absence of fat involvement by radiologic criteria. Preoperative full extraocular motility correlates well with the likelihood of preserving orbit function, but it, too, is not a perfect prognosticator. To complicate the matter further, there may be times when tumor does extend intraorbitally to involve orbital fat focally, but orbit preservation remains a viable option. Evaluating this option is an individual judgment decision by the surgeon in conjunction with the radiation oncologist and the patient. If a close decision is anticipated, it is often best to make this decision late in the surgical procedure, after frozen-section assessment of other key potential margins such as dura, lateral sphenoid sinus, and posterior orbital periosteum. If close or microscopically positive margins are inevitable at other locations, and the eye was functional preoperatively (Fig. 8), the surgeon must decide whether exenteration would materially improve the prognosis or significantly facilitate postoperative radiation treatment.

*What are the options for dural repair and management of potential cerebrospinal leakage?*

If a bifrontal craniotomy is part of the surgical procedure, a pericranial galeal flap is highly successful in managing potential CSF leaks and in

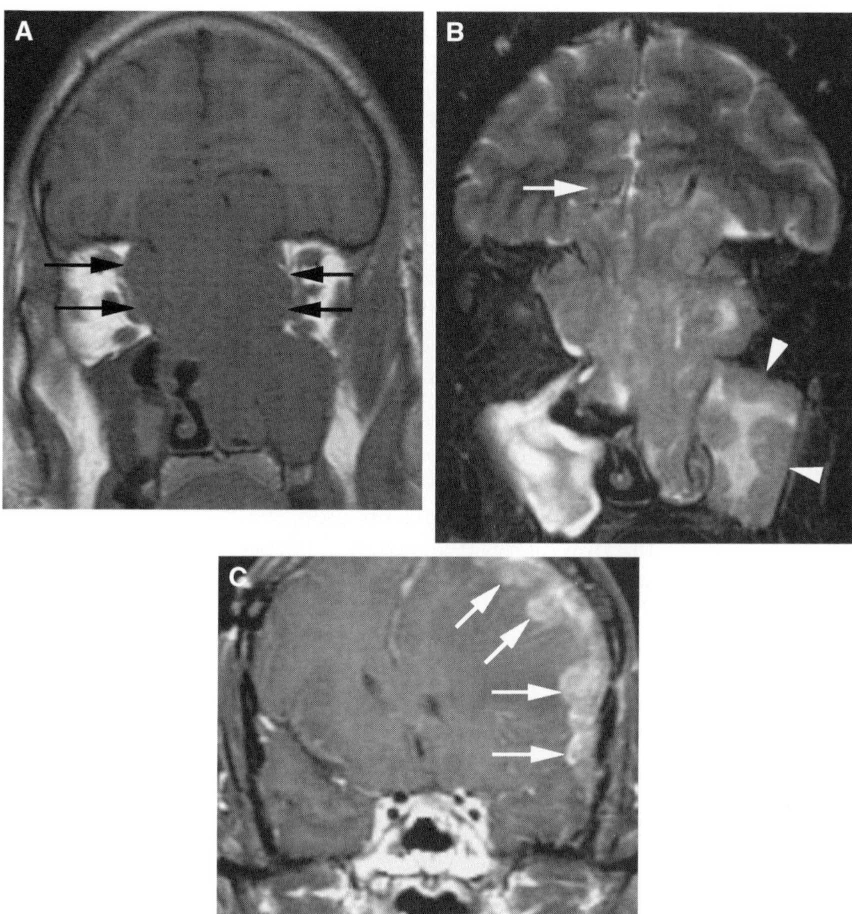

Fig. 8. A 27-year-old man with extensive sinonasal undifferentiated carcinoma presented for evaluation of treatment options. (*A*) A coronal T1-weighted image demonstrates a large mass filling the nasal cavity and the ethmoid and left maxillary sinuses and extending into the anterior cranial fossa. Although gross tumor is seen penetrating the lamina papyraceae bilaterally (*black arrows*), the orbital fat is not definitely abnormal, and the involvement may be only subperiosteal. (*B*) A coronal fast spin echo T2-weighted image demonstrates the intermediate signal intensity of this highly cellular tumor, which has infiltrated throughout the submucosa of the left maxillary sinus (*white arrowheads*). A small focus of T2 hyperintensity in the right frontal lobe (*white arrow*) is concerning for brain edema caused by tumor invasion. At surgery minimal brain involvement was noted, and the orbits were preserved because the closest margin of resection was clearly intracranial. Full extraocular motility and normal vision were maintained. The patient received postoperative IMRT and chemotherapy. (*C*) Seven months later, the patient developed progressive headaches. A coronal postgadolinium T1-weighted image with fat saturation demonstrates extensive infiltration of the dura with tumor (*arrows*), with underlying brain edema and subfalcial brain herniation.

segregating the sterile intracranial cavity from the bacteria-laden paranasal sinuses. It is usually advantageous to repair any dural defect directly using any of a number of options such as temporalis fascia, bovine pericardium, or fascia lata.

It has been established that endoscopic repair of CSF leaks is highly successful. Hence, for limited dissections at the skull base in which a craniotomy is not done (or a pericranial flap is not available), it is possible to reconstruct the defect using autologous free tissue, such as a mucosal graft, rather than the standard pericranial galeal flap that is generally available with a bifrontal craniotomy.

## How should the frontal sinus be managed?

The best way to prevent a possible late complication of frontal sinus mucocele is to ensure that all areas of the frontal sinus can drain into the ethmoid sinuses. If the frontal sinus is entered as part of the frontal craniotomy, and a pericranial galeal flap is used, it is necessary to remove the mucosa from the now-segregated superior portion of the frontal sinus and also to bur away 1 to 2 mm of the surface as one would as part of a frontal sinus obliteration. Fat obliteration or removal of the posterior table may at times be indicated to prevent a mucocele or to augment management of a CSF leak.

Occasionally, epidural air may fill the frontal fossa postoperatively, particularly if a dehydrated, CSF-depleted brain does not fully re-expand. Excessive drainage of lumbar CSF can contribute to this condition. If a CSF leak has been excluded as the source of the extradural air, it is likely that nasally inspired air is accessing the extradural space through the superior ethmoid or frontal sinus surgical defect. Intubation and maintaining an inflated endotracheal cuff for several days usually facilitates resolution of the problem. If the air persists, a tracheotomy may be indicated, as well as careful reassessment to be sure there is not an occult CSF leak.

## When is supplemental bony reconstruction of the anterior skull base indicated?

Smith and Ducic [38] reviewed nicely the anatomy and versatility of extended pericranial flaps for closure of the anterior skull base. Pericranial or pericranial-galeal flaps, usually anteriorly based but sometimes laterally based, are vascularized pieces of tissue positioned and sealed in a water-tight manner so that they prevent CSF leakage and segregate the brain from the contaminated paranasal sinus flora. They also eliminate dead space and serve as a sling to support the brain, preventing frontal lobe herniation.

In some cases, however, reconstruction of large anterior skull base defects may benefit from adding split calvarial bone from the inner table of the craniotomy flap to support the brain further, preventing herniation and oscillopsia or pulsatile exophthalmos if the orbital roof has been removed.

Large defects (greater than 3 to 4 cm both in anterior-posterior and transverse directions) typically include the orbital roof and part of the planum sphenoidale [39]. The split calvarial bone is placed superior to the pericranial flap, and the distal part of the soft tissue flap is reflected back over the bone to enclose it fully within soft tissue.

*How long postoperatively should a lumbar subarachnoid drain be used in an effort to reduce the likelihood of a persistent cerebrospinal leak?*

One of the parameters to be considered in determining the best surgical approach is minimizing brain retraction. If CSF decompression would reduce the risk of brain retraction, it should be used intraoperatively. But does a lumbar drain used postoperatively reduce the likelihood of a CSF leak? Certainly, permanent shunting using a lumboperitoneal (or similar) shunt for a recalcitrant CSF leak that cannot be repaired seems to be effective, and a drain for 3 to 5 days postoperatively (or following trauma) is widely used. Convincing data that a drain used for a few days is beneficial are lacking, however, and some centers have curtailed its use because of the potential complications associated with overdrainage of fluid. These complications include infection and promoting pneumocephalus, particularly herniation-inducing pneumocephalus.

## Complications

Complications have become less frequent as increased experience has been gained with anterior skull base surgery. Although the rate of all complications, major and minor, is about 35%, the rate of complications with long-term consequences is less than 4% to 5% in most series. Operative mortality is well under 1%; the authors have had no operative deaths in more than a decade. The incidence of CSF leaks is less than 2%, as is the incidence of meningitis or brain abscess. CSF leaks have been addressed with re-repair (and the rare ventriculoperitoneal shunt). Infectious complications have resolved with antibiotics or surgical drainage. Serious central nervous system deficits (including cerebrovascular accidents, unanticipated blindness, postinfection deficits, and autonomic dysfunction) have occurred in only 2% to 3% of patients. Loss of the anterior bone flap secondary to osteomyelitis, once a serious problem in anterior skull base surgery, has not occurred in a decade. Nor have the authors seen intracranial bleeds or hematomas. Pericranial-galeal flaps and, for larger defects and for patients who have undergone prior irradiation, microvascular free flaps [40] have contributed greatly to the reduced incidence of postoperative CSF leaks and wound or bone infections. The authors believe that they have seen less frontal lobe encephalomalacia because they have tailored approaches to minimize the need for brain retraction. Finally, medical complications such as pneumonias, arrhythmias, and, rarely, myocardial infarctions have been steady at 10%, sometimes extending hospitalizations but usually not leading to death.

## Radiation therapy

A major impetus to the development of anterior cranial base surgery was the disappointing results of irradiation with or without the surgery of the time for tumors that extended to the skull base. Numerous series showed no better than 50% (and in most series 25% to 35%) survival for the more common malignancies [41–43]. Planning radiation fields near the brain, optic nerves, and optic chiasm is challenging [44]. The ocular lens can tolerate about 50 Gy. Above this level, cataracts develop, but they are treatable. In the optic nerve and chiasm, there is a 10% incidence of optic neuritis if the dose received is 50 to 55 Gy, but the incidence increases to 20% for doses above 65 Gy. Minimal radionecrosis of the inferior portions of the frontal lobe is often—but not always—tolerated with a minimum of long-term symptoms, but in some cases radionecrosis of the brain may lead to severe cerebral edema, brain herniation, and death. Although there is variation in the literature regarding the dose of radiation that should be given to the gross target volume, most centers aim for a minimum of 60 Gy, with many centers advocating a minimum of 65 Gy or more.

Before the development of IMRT, charged particles were often used when irradiating the anterior skull base. The rapid falloff in dose afforded by protons permitted, for example, a dose of 60 to 80 Gy to be administered to clival chordomas without undue risk to the optic nerves and chiasm. Proton beam irradiation is available at only a few centers, notably Harvard and Loma Linda University. Preliminary experience with proton IMRT may offer even tighter fields than conventional IMRT, allowing more of a tumor to receive adequate doses safely.

## Chemotherapy

Concomitant postoperative chemotherapy [45] and radiation therapy are indicated for SCC of the paranasal sinuses. For lymphoma, chemotherapy is usually the mainstay of treatment, depending on the specific histologic type of lymphoma and the stage of disease. For esthesioneuroblastoma, the role of chemotherapy is controversial: some recommend it for all Kadish C lesions, but others reserve it for extensive tumors with intradural extension. For high-grade neuroendocrine carcinomas and sinonasal undifferentiated carcinomas, cisplatin and VP-16 are often considered. Specific regimens for a particular tumor histology depend on the overall health and tolerance of the patient.

## Results of anterior skull base surgery plus irradiation

Many series from different centers, including Stanford Medical Center, have documented encouraging local control rates compared with historic results that do not include skull base resection for a number of malignant histologies (including esthesioneuroblastoma, adenoid cystic carcinoma, adenocarcinoma, and SCC). A summary of these data, with 5-year survival rates, is provided in Box 1 [46–55].

Esthesioneuroblastomas and adenocarcinomas generally do best, with 5-year survivals approaching or exceeding 80%. A number of tumors are in the middle range with 5-year survivals of approximately 50% to 60%. Melanoma and sinonasal undifferentiated tumors do much more poorly, and treatment strategies for patients with these two histologies should stress functional preservation and the need for multicenter trials to attempt to elucidate how best to incorporate chemotherapy and IMRT or possibly proton IMRT into the management of these patients.

## Treatment of recurrent disease

*Perineural spread to Meckel's cave and the cavernous sinus*

Perineural spread along V2 (or V1) is especially common in SCC and adenoid cystic carcinoma but may occur with other histologies. New dysesthesia or anesthesia, with or without pain, along the lateral nose and maxillary alveolar ridge (V2) or above the eye (V1) warrants an MRI. The MRI must be done with meticulous attention to the skull base and cavernous sinuses, because imaging findings may be subtle and are often overlooked. Spread from V to VII may occur by a number of routes, such as the auriculotemporal nerve or the greater superficial petrosal nerve, and this possibility should be carefully assessed in any patient with a history of paranasal sinus malignancy and a new facial palsy. Radiosurgery has been

---

**Box 1. Histology and 5-year survival (%)**

Esthesioneuroblastoma: 62%–95% (most, 80%–95%)
Adenocarcinoma meta-analysis: 78%
Adenoid cystic carcinoma: 40%–60%; an additional 15%–20% alive with disease
Sarcomas: 50%–60%; an additional 20% alive with disease
SCC meta-analysis (including skin with perineural spread): 60%
Melanoma meta-analysis: 23%
Sinonasal undifferentiated carcinoma: less than 1%–15%

used in perineural extension of tumor both to control pain and to retard tumor growth, with pain relief often occurring in about 6 months and with a 40% rate of clinical or radiologic 5-year durable response in controlling tumor progression.

## Neck metastases

Neck metastases occur about 20% of cases of SCC of the paranasal sinuses and in about 10% of esthesioneuroblastomas. If the primary site is controlled, a neck dissection is indicated, with postoperative irradiation if there has not already been neck irradiation. When there has been prior neck irradiation, there may be a role for intraoperative radiation therapy at the time of the neck dissection [56].

## Local recurrence

Treatment of paranasal sinus malignancies that recur locally is usually limited by prior irradiation and prior surgery. In addition, a tumor that has demonstrated recurrence may be relatively radiation-resistant and chemo-therapy-resistant. Depending on the histology, there may be chemotherapy protocols or combined chemotherapy and re-irradiation protocols that are of some value. Depending on current symptoms and extent of recurrence, there may be a role for palliative surgery.

## Summary

Anterior skull base surgery has evolved significantly over the past 50 years, moving from early experimental attempts to improve dismal control rates associated with a high incidence of life-threatening complications to a well-accepted multidisciplinary subspecialty with proven improved results. Further reduction in perioperative side effects, decreased length of hospital stay, and improved aesthetic results are ongoing goals of the discipline. Modified surgical approaches are constantly under development and review. The standard by which these modifications will be judged remains a bifrontal craniotomy with or without a supraorbital rim approach and with or without a well-camouflaged transfacial extended external ethmoidectomy incision without a lateral rhinotomy. At times endoscopic-assisted approaches provide the visualization that allows foregoing a facial incision, and endoscopic techniques will continue to evolve and disseminate. Selected highly experienced centers are exploring the increased use of endoscopic resections without craniotomy, demonstrating that this approach is feasible for highly selected tumors. A subfrontal approach with minimal brain retraction is occasionally ideal when frontal bone and nasal bone must be removed because of tumor involvement.

Effective skull base surgery requires an established multidisciplinary team that involves otolaryngologist-head and neck surgeons, neurosurgeons, plastic surgeons, neuroradiologists, medical oncologists, radiation oncologists, prosthodontists, and other supporting physicians and allied health professionals. Guided by local experience and influenced by a variety of patient and physician factors, this group should cooperatively choose which set of approaches and its variations seems most appropriate for each individual patient.

## References


[1] Smith RR, Klopp CT, Williams JM. Surgical treatment of cancer of the frontal sinus and adjacent areas. Cancer 1954;7:991–4.

[2] Dandy WE. Orbital tumor: results following the transcranial operative attack. New York: Oskar Priest; 1941.

[3] Rae BS, McLean JM. Combined intracranial and orbital operation for retinoblastoma. Arch Ophthalmol 1943;30:437–45.

[4] Ketcham AS, Wilkins RH, Van Buren JM, et al. A combined intracranial approach to the paranasal sinuses. Am J Surg 1963;106:698–703.

[5] Van Buren JM, Ommaya AK, Ketcham AS. Ten years' experience with radical combined craniofacial resection of malignant tumors of the paranasal sinuses. J Neurosurg 1968;28: 341–50.

[6] Kaplan MJ, McDermott MW, Gutin PH, et al. Transcutaneous transfacial approaches to the anterior skull base. In: Lawton M, editor. Operative techniques in neurosurgery 2000;3:53–6.

[7] Har-El G. Anterior craniofacial resection without facial skin incision—a review. Otolaryngol Head Neck Surg 2004;130:780–7.

[8] Patel SG, Singh B, Polluri A, et al. Craniofacial surgery for malignant skull base tumors: report of an international collaborative study. Cancer 2003;98:1179–87.

[8a] Lang DA. Surgery of the cranial base. In: Sekhar LN, Janecka IP, editors. Surgery of Cranial Base Tumors. New York: Raven Press; 1993. p. 93–121.

[9] Jho HD, Ha HG. Endoscopic endonasal skull base surgery: Part 1—the midline anterior fossa skull base. Minim Invasive Neurosurg 2004;47:1–8.

[10] Tiwari R, van der Wal J, van der Waal I, et al. Studies of the anatomy and pathology of the orbit in carcinoma of the maxillary sinus and their impact on preservation of the eye in maxillectomy. Head Neck 1998;20(3):193–6.

[11] Fee WE Jr, Moir MS, Choi EC, et al. Nasopharyngectomy for recurrent nasopharyngeal cancer: a 2- to 17-year follow-up. Arch Otolaryngol Head Neck Surg 2002;128(3):280–4.

[12] Ibrahim HZ, Moir MS, Fee WW. Nasopharyngectomy after failure of 2 courses of radiation therapy. Arch Otolaryngol Head Neck Surg 2002;128:1196–7.

[13] To EW, Yuen EH, Tsang WM, et al. The use of stereotactic navigation guidance in minimally invasive transnasal nasopharyngectomy: a comparison with the conventional open transfacial approach. Br J Radiol 2002;75(892):345–50.

[14] To EW, Lai EC, Cheng JH, et al. Nasopharyngectomy for recurrent nasopharyngeal carcinoma: a review of 31 patients and prognostic factors. Laryngoscope 2002;112:1877–82.

[15] Myers LL, Oxford LE. Differential diagnosis and treatment options in paranasal sinus cancer. Surg Oncol Clin N Am 2004;13:167–86.

[16] Bentz BG, Bilsky MH, Shah JP, et al. Anterior skull base surgery for malignant tumors: a multivariate analysis of 27 years of experience. Head Neck 2003;25:515–20.

[17] Le QT, Fu KK, Kaplan MJ, et al. Lymph node metastasis in maxillary sinus carcinoma. Int J Radiat Oncol Biol Phys 2000;46(3):541–9.

[18] Paulino AC, Fisher SG, Marks JE. Is prophylactic neck irradiation indicated in patients with squamous cell carcinoma of the maxillary sinus? Int J Radiat Oncol Biol Phys 1997;39(2): 283–9.

[19] Pitman KT, Prokopakis EP, Aydogan B, et al. The role of skull base surgery for the treatment of adenoid cystic carcinoma of the sinonasal tract. Head Neck 1999;21(5):402–7.

[20] Dias FL, Sa GM, Lima RA, et al. Patterns of failure and outcome in esthesioneuroblastoma. Arch Otolaryngol Head Neck Surg 2003;129:1186–92.

[21] Bradley PJ, Jones NS, Robertson I. Diagnosis and management of esthesioneuroblastoma. Curr Opin Otolaryngol Head Neck Surg 2003;11:112–8.

[22] Lund VJ, Howard D, Wei W, et al. Olfactory neuroblastoma: past, present, and future? Laryngoscope 2003;113:502–7.

[23] Brandwein MS, Rothstein A, Lawson W, et al. Sinonasal melanoma. A clinicopathological study of 25 cases and literature meta-analysis. Arch Otolaryngol Head Neck Surg 1997;123: 290–6.

[24] Patel SG, Prasad ML, Escrig M, et al. Primary mucosal malignant melanoma of the head and neck. Head Neck 2002;24:247–57.

[25] Kramer D, Durham JS, Sheehan F, et al. Sinonasal undifferentiated carcinoma: case series and systematic review of the literature. J Otolaryngol 2004;33:32–6.

[26] Kim BS, Vongtama R, Juillard G. Sinonasal undifferentiated carcinoma: case series and literature review. Am J Otolaryngol 2004;25:162–6.

[27] Chan AW, Pommier P, Deschler DG, et al. Combined proton radiotherapy with chemotherapy for advanced sinonasal neuroendocrine carcinoma [abstract]. Proceedings of the Sixth International Conference on Head and Neck Cancer. Washington, D.C., 2004. p. 293.

[28] Har-El G. Anterior craniofacial resection without facial skin incisions—a review. Otolaryngol Head Neck Surg 2004;103:780–7.

[29] Thaler ER, Kotapka M, Lanza DC, et al. Endoscopically assisted anterior cranial skull base resection of sinonasal tumors. Am J Rhinol 1999;13:303–10.

[30] Yuen APW, Fung CT, Hung KN. Endoscopic cranionasal resection of anterior skull base tumor. Am J Otolaryngol 1997;18:431–3.

[31] Har-El G, Todor R. Anterior craniofacial resection without facial skin incisions. Skull Base 2003;13(Suppl 1):13–20.

[32] Fagan JJ, Snyderman CH, Carrau RL, et al. Nasopharyngeal angiofibromas: selecting a surgical approach. Head Neck 1997;19:391–9.

[33] Carrau RL, Snyderman CH, Kassam AB, et al. Endoscopic and endoscopic-assisted surgery for juvenile angiofibroma. Laryngoscope 2001;111:483–7.

[34] Al-Nashar IS, Carrau RL, Herrera A, et al. Endoscopic transnasal transpterygopalatine fossa approach to the lateral recess of the sphenoid sinus. Laryngoscope 2004;114:528–32.

[35] Raveh J, Laedrach K, Speiser M, et al. The subcranial approach for fronto-orbital and antero-posterior skull base tumors. Arch Otolaryngol Head Neck Surg 1993;119:382–93.

[36] Cocke EW, Robertson JH. Extended unilateral maxillotomy approach. In: Donald PJ, editor. Surgery of the skull base. Philadelphia: Lippincott-Raven; 1998. p. 207–37.

[37] Casiano RR, Numa WA, Falquez AM. Endoscopic resection of esthesioneuroblastoma. Am J Rhinol 2001;15:271–9.

[38] Smith JE, Ducuc Y. The versatile extended pericranial flap for closure of skull base defects. Otolaryngol Head Neck Surg 2004;130:704–11.

[39] Rodrigues M, O'Malley BW, Staecker H, et al. Extended pericranial flap and bone graft reconstruction in anterior skull base surgery. Otolaryngol Head Neck Surg 2004;131:69–76.

[40] Clayman GL, DeMonte F, Jaffe DM, et al. Outcome and complications of extended cranial-base resection requiring microvascular free-tissue transfer. Arch Otolaryngol Head Neck Surg 1995;121:1253–7.

[41] Adams EJ, Nutting CM, Convery DJ, et al. Potential role of intensity-modulated radiotherapy in the treatment of tumors of the maxillary sinus. Int J Radiat Oncol Biol Phys 2001;51(3):579–88.

[42] Remouchamps V, Van Duyse B, Vakaet L, et al. An implementation strategy for IMRT of ethmoid sinus cancer with bilateral sparing of the optic pathways. Int J Radiat Oncol Biol Phys 2001;51(2):318–31.

[43] Waldron JN, O'Sullivan B, Gullane P, et al. Carcinoma of the maxillary antrum: a retrospective analysis of 110 cases. Radiother Oncol 2000;57(2):167–73.

[44] Rasch C, Eisbruch A, Remeijer P, et al. Irradiation of paranasal sinus tumors, a delineation and dose comparison study. Int J Radiat Oncol Biol Phys 2002;52(1):120–7.

[45] Diaz EM Jr, Kies MS. Chemotherapy for skull base cancers. Otolaryngol Clin North Am 2001;34(6):1079–85, viii.

[46] Janecka IP, Sen C, Sekhar LN, et al. Cranial base surgery: results in 183 patients. Otolaryngol Head Neck Surg 1994;110(6):539–46.

[47] Janecka IP, Sen C, Sekhar L, et al. Treatment of paranasal sinus cancer with cranial base surgery: results. Laryngoscope 1994;104(5 Pt 1):553–5.

[48] Irish JC, Gullane PJ, Gentili F, et al. Tumors of the skull base: outcome and survival analysis of 77 cases. Head Neck 1994;16(1):3–10.

[49] O'Malley BW Jr, Janecka IP. Evolution of outcomes in cranial base surgery. Semin Surg Oncol 1995;11(3):221–7.

[50] McCaffrey TV, Olsen KD, Yohanan JM, et al. Factors affecting survival of patients with tumors of the anterior skull base. Laryngoscope 1994;104(8 Pt 1):940–5.

[51] Boyle JO, Shah KC, Shah JP. Craniofacial resection for malignant neoplasms of the skull base: an overview. J Surg Oncol 1998;69:275–84.

[52] Shah JP, Kraus DH, Arbit E, et al. Craniofacial resection for tumors involving the anterior skull base. Otolaryngol Head Neck Surg 1992;106:387–93.

[53] Harbo G, Grau C, Bundgaard T, et al. Cancer of the nasal cavity and paranasal sinuses. A clinico-pathological study of 277 patients. Acta Oncol 1997;36(1):45–50.

[54] Lund VJ, Howard DJ, Wei WI, et al. Craniofacial resection for tumors of the nasal cavity and paranasal sinuses—a 17-year experience. Head Neck 1998;20(2):97–105.

[55] Dulguerov P, Jacobsen MS, Allal AS, et al. Nasal and paranasal sinus carcinoma: are we making progress? A series of 220 patients and a systematic review. Cancer 2001;92(12): 3012–29.

[56] Coleman CW, Roach M III, Ling SM, et al. Adjuvant electron-beam IORT in high-risk head and neck cancer patients. Front Radiat Ther Oncol 1997;31:105–11.

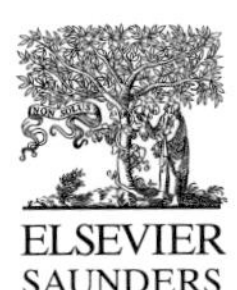

ELSEVIER
SAUNDERS

Otolaryngol Clin N Am
38 (2005) 133–144

OTOLARYNGOLOGIC
CLINICS
OF NORTH AMERICA

# Endoscopic Management of Anterior Skull Base Tumors

Gady Har-El, MD, FACS[a,b],*,
Roy R. Casiano, MD, FACS[c]

[a]*Departments of Otolaryngology and Neurosurgery,
State University of New York-Downstate Medical Center, New York, NY, USA*
[b]*Continuum Cancer Centers, New York, NY, USA*
[c]*Department of Otolaryngology, University of Miami School of Medicine,
Miami, FL, USA*

Skull base surgery, in general, and anterior skull base surgery, in particular, are relatively young disciplines within otolaryngology-head and neck surgery. Within this new frontier in head and neck oncology, anterior craniofacial resection (ACFR) has become a standard procedure for management of lesions of the anterior cranial base. A review of the progress in head and neck oncologic surgery during the last 40 years shows that ACFR is probably one of the few surgical extirpative procedures that expanded the ability to remove tumors and increase cure rates. Most of the other novel surgical procedures in head and neck surgery were introduced to increase anatomic and functional preservation and to improve reconstruction, but rarely do they increase extirpative abilities.

The history of anterior skull base surgery and ACFR has been reviewed by Donald [1]. In 1941, Dandy [2] described resection of an orbital tumor by means of anterior craniotomy, which included entering the ethmoid complex. This report was followed by Rae and McClean [3], who used a combined transorbital-transcranial approach, and by Smith et al [4] who performed a combined transfacial-transcranial approach for tumor removal. ACFR as introduced by Ketcham et al [5] has become the standard procedure for management of lesions of the anterior skull base. In fact, the classic ACFR performed today includes the same facial skin incisions combined with a bicoronal incision and the same bony cuts described by

* Corresponding author. Department of Otolaryngology, Long Island College Hospital, 134 Atlantic Avenue, Brooklyn, NY 11201.
*E-mail address:* gadyh@aol.com (G. Har-El).

0030-6665/05/$ - see front matter © 2005 Elsevier Inc. All rights reserved.
doi:10.1016/j.otc.2004.09.007 *oto.theclinics.com*

Ketcham [5]. ACFR has been shown to have a positive impact on treatment results of paranasal sinus tumors extending to the anterior skull base [6,7].

During the last 2 decades, modifications of ACFR have been reported. Some surgeons extended the exposure and expanded tumor resection abilities (eg, orbitocranial approaches, combined anterior/middle fossa approaches), whereas others described procedures to reduce complication rates, preserve function (eg, vision, smell), improve reconstruction, and improve cosmesis [8–10].

With the introduction of endoscopic sinus techniques and instrumentation, surgeons have begun to use endoscopic approaches for management of anterior skull base lesions [11–18]. Recent advances in computer-assisted surgery stimulated surgeons to expand the indications for endoscopic surgery while preserving safety. The increased popularity of endoscopic techniques did not come without debate and controversy. Many surgeons believe that these procedures may compromise the ability to remove tumor completely. Others argue that, when possible, complete en bloc tumor removal is essential. It has been repeatedly shown that positive surgical margins at the first extirpative procedure have a strong negative impact on outcome and overall survival [7]. Other surgeons argue that even open procedures do not necessarily provide en bloc resection in this complicated three-dimensional anatomic region, and that piecemeal removal does not reduce control rates as long as complete removal of the tumor is achieved at the end of the procedure. Before discussing the controversies, this article describes a few endoscopic variants of ACFR.

## Endoscopic-assisted anterior craniofacial resection

For tumors without significant inferior extension (ie, without involvement of the nasal floor) and for tumors without significant lateral extension (ie, without extension of the tumor into the maxillary sinus), transnasal endoscopes may be used to assist with ACFR, which is done transcranially. The procedure begins with intracranial exposure through either a conventional frontal craniotomy or the subcranial approach. With this procedure, actual tumor removal is not done endoscopically [8,10]. Osteotomes or other instruments passed from the cranial side of the skull base into the nasal cavity or the ethmoid complex are guided with the help of transnasal endoscopes (Fig. 1). The orientation and direction of a lateral ethmoid entry or posterior and anterior septal cuts and their relations to the tumor can be assessed endoscopically. This assessment can ensure safe margins around the tumor. Also, certain inferior cuts such as inferior nasal septal cut or lateral nasal (medial maxillary wall) cuts can be performed through the nose with the help of the endoscopes. For many tumors, complete en bloc removal of the tumor specimen can be achieved. The tumor is removed from the cranial side of the skull base.

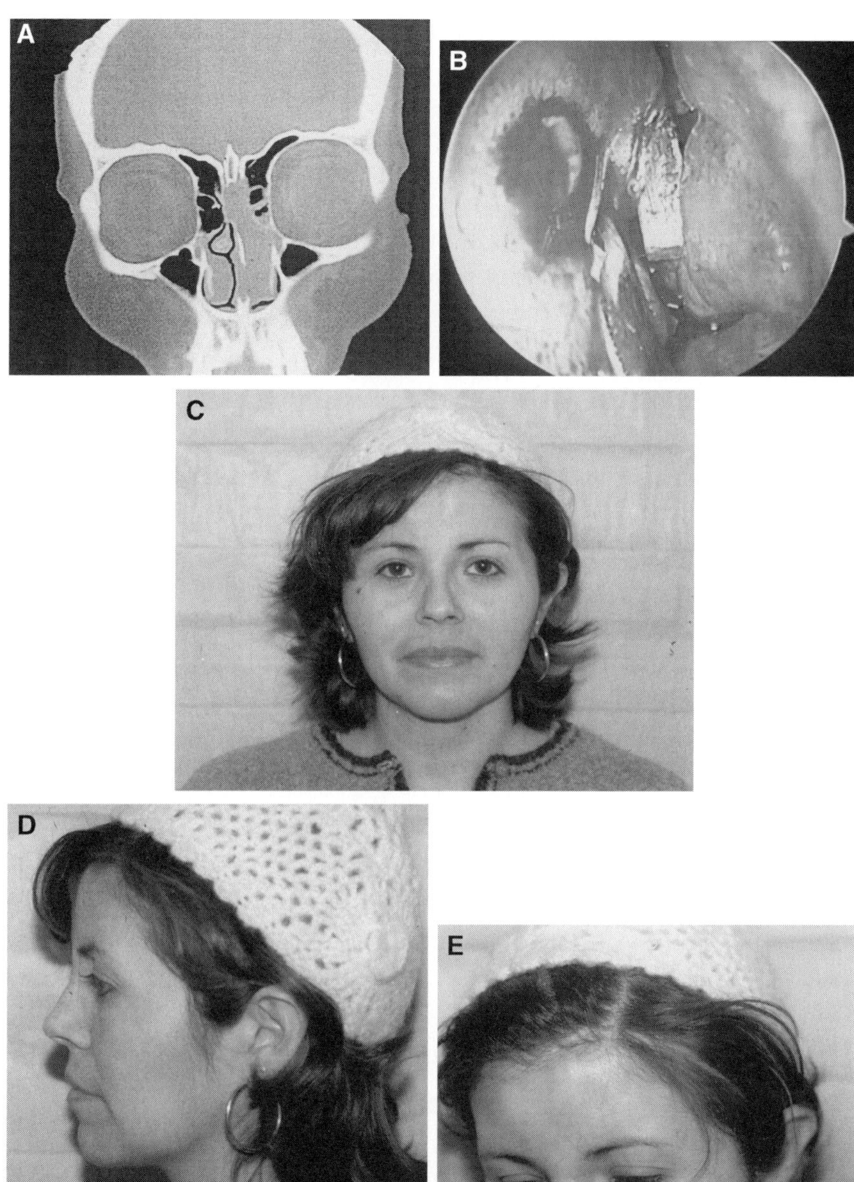

Fig. 1. Endoscopic-assisted ACFR for esthesioneuroblastoma. (*A*) Preoperative coronal CT. (*B*) Endoscopic guidance of osteotome placed through the craniotomy. (*C*) Frontal view 3 years after surgery. (*D*) Lateral view 3 years after surgery. (*E*) Hidden coronal incision. (*From* Har-El G. Anterior craniofacial resection without facial skin incisions. Otolaryngol Head Neck Surg 2004;130:780–7; with permission.)

## Endoscopic anterior craniofacial resection without craniotomy

Endoscopic anterior craniofacial resection without craniotomy was described by Casiano (Fig. 2) [17,18]. He reported good results with its application for management of esthesioneuroblastoma. The procedure begins with endoscopic transnasal debulking of the tumor with a 4-mm microdebrider. The nasal septum, lateral nasal wall, and posterior choanae are exposed. The remaining parts of the procedure are performed principally with nonbiting forceps to assure adequate mucosal stripping and to yield tissue for pathologic analysis and mapping. A suction filter/collector (sock) is used for each side to collect the tissue debris removed by the microdebrider.

Endoscopic medial maxillectomy is performed if the tumor involves the ethmoid sinus. It includes removal of the ipsilateral inferior and middle turbinates, medial maxillary wall with the nasolacrimal duct, total ethmoidectomy without mucosal preservation, removal of the lamina

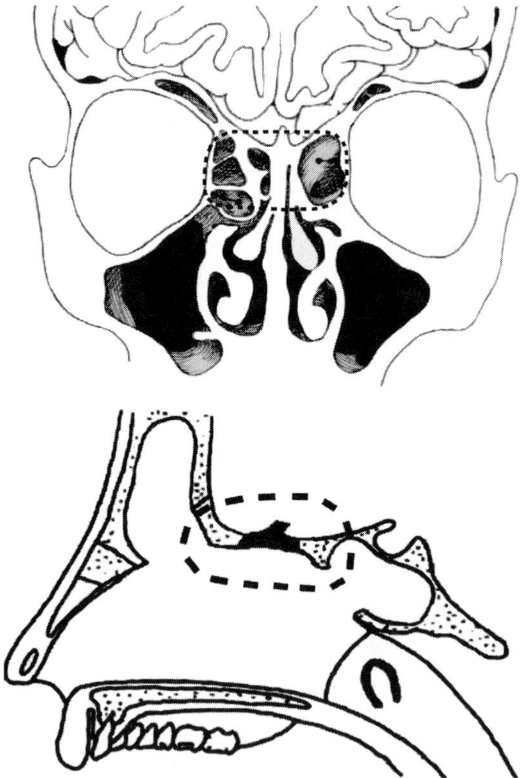

Fig. 2. Bilateral endoscopic anterior skull base resection. Dotted line displays the minimal resection margins in the coronal (*upper picture*) and sagittal (*lower picture*) planes. Additional resection may include a medial maxillectomy and septectomy.

papyracea throughout the length of the ethmoid cavity, and wide sphenoid and frontal sinusotomies. Total ethmoidectomy and middle meatal antrostomies are also performed on the contralateral side if the tumor extends beyond the olfactory cleft on the ipsilateral side or if there is radiologic evidence of contralateral disease.

The superior nasal septum is removed back to uninvolved margins, creating a space to allow the surgeon to work through both nostrils. A complete septectomy may be necessary. The sphenopalatine foramina are identified and cauterized bilaterally. An additional suction is used to maintain the nasopharynx clear of blood and debris. The anterior skull base resection and extended frontal sinusotomy (modified Lothrop procedure) begins. This approach exposes the anterior margin of resection. Large cutting burrs are used to thin down the bone at the nasofrontal suture line (nasion) and to enlarge the common frontal sinusotomy, exposing the posterior frontal sinus wall. At the posterior end of resection, a wide bilateral sphenoid sinusotomy is performed by removing the rostrum and intersinus septum. The optic nerves and carotid arteries are identified bilaterally but are left undisturbed. The fovea ethmoidalis and sphenoid roof anterior to the optic chiasm are thinned with large burrs to an eggshell thickness and are removed with rongeurs to exposed the underlying dura circumferentially around the remaining bony septum, middle turbinate remnants, and the olfactory cleft bilaterally. The dura is elevated off the orbital roof laterally to facilitate placement of graft reconstruction at the end of the procedure. The anterior and posterior ethmoidal arteries are cauterized with a bipolar cautery. Adherence of the dura to the orbital roof may signify a more extensive tumor invasion, potentially necessitating an open neurosurgical approach.

Dural resection begins at the posterior frontal region, extending posteriorly to the optic chiasm. Laterally, the dural margin is initially resected a few millimeters medial to the junction of the orbital wall and the ethmoid roof. En bloc removal of the entire specimen is done in an anterior-to-posterior direction. The specimen includes the dura, bilateral cribriform plates with olfactory bulbs, middle turbinate remnants, perpendicular plate of the septum, and the inferior aspect of the crista galli (Fig. 3). This removal allows direct visualization, access to any vessels adjacent to these structures, and avoidance of undue trauma to any cortical vessels or brain parenchyma. Bipolar cautery is used to control any bleeding vessels. Adjacent brain parenchyma and the intracranial cavity are inspected for presence of neoplasm, and frozen-section diagnosis of specimens from the dural margins, olfactory nerve endings, septum, and nasopharynx are obtained. Smaller unilateral lesions are resected in a similar fashion but with sparing of the contralateral septal mucosa, cribriform plate, and sinuses. At the conclusion of the procedure, there are approximately 15 to 20 specimen cups from separate anatomic areas (right and left anterior ethmoid, posterior ethmoid, sphenoid, medial maxillary wall, maxillary sinuses,

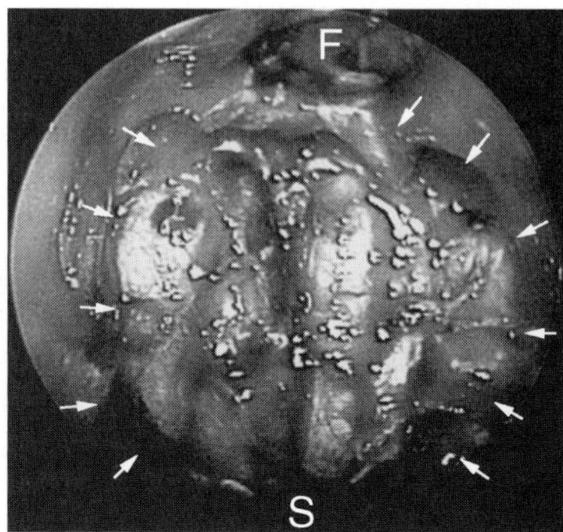



Fig. 3. Endoscopic view of the anterior skull base defect with a 70° telescope. Small arrows demarcate the orbital margins. The extended frontal (*F*) and sphenoid (*S*) cavities make up the anterior and posterior margins of resection, respectively.

turbinates, septum, frontal recess, and nasopharynx, among others.). These specimens allow accurate pathologic mapping of the tumor. At the conclusion of the procedure, endoscopic marsupialization of the lacrimal sac is performed with the microdebrider to minimize the chance of stenosis and epiphora.

## Reconstruction

The extent of reconstruction depends on the size of the defect. Larger defects require a composite repair with a two- to three-ply lyophilized dura or a thick alloderm. This graft material acts merely as a scaffold for ingrowth of granulations and fibroblasts. Crusting and secondary healing with granulation will occur over the next 8 to 12 months, but it is usually left undisturbed. If a lyophilized dura is used, the surgeon should ascertain that the facility has been approved by the Food and Drug Administration and the donors were tested for the presence of slow viruses or other potentially communicable diseases. For larger defects extending the full length of the anterior skull base (approximately, 2 × 3 cm), the lyophilized dura is tucked for at least 1 cm circumferentially between the remaining dura and the orbital roof. For a smaller defect, a variety of reconstructive techniques are available. An intranasal mucoperichondrial graft is placed firmly around the margins of the skull base defect (on the nasal side over the orbital wall, superior sphenoid sinus, and inferior posterior wall of the frontal sinus), with half of the graft over viable tissue and the other half over lyophilized dura. The graft is obtained from the remaining normal contralateral inferior turbinate. A separate alloderm sheet may be used for this purpose (Fig. 4). The mucosal graft is held tightly in place with absorbable gelatin sponge

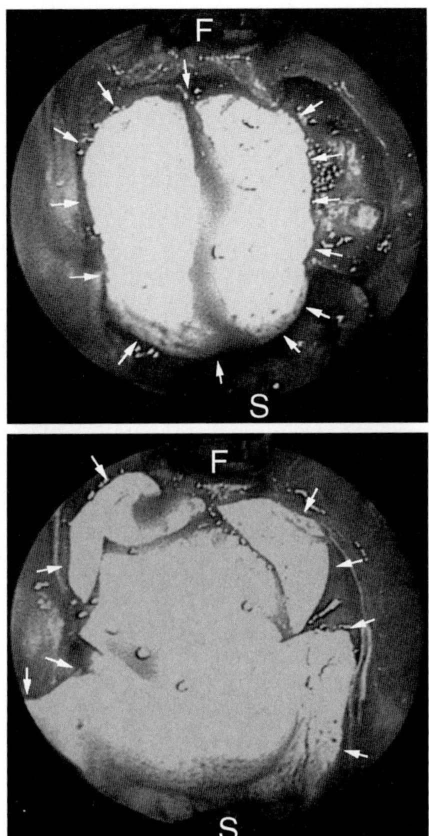



Fig. 4. Endoscopic view of anterior skull base reconstruction with acellular dermis. Small arrows demarcate the orbital wall. The extended frontal (*F*) and sphenoid (*S*) cavities are noted. The upper picture illustrates the intracranial portion of the repair with a sheet of alloderm tucked intracranially over the orbital roof and sphenoid planum and behind the posterior wall of the frontal sinus bilaterally. The lower picture shows the intranasal portion of the repair with an onlay sheet of alloderm over the previous repair as well as the medial orbital wall, superiorly.

(Gelfoam) and Merocel tampons (Merocel Corp., Mystic, CT). The tampons are removed within 7 days for large defects or 5 days for small defects. Lumbar drains are not used. Patients are discharged home, taking stool softeners and antibiotics, after 4 to 5 days. Postoperatively, all patients undergoing primary resection receive adjuvant radiotherapy beginning approximately 5 weeks after surgery.

## Endoscopic craniofacial resection

Different variations of this procedure have been described in the literature [11–16]. Endoscopic ACFR includes transnasal endoscopic management of the lesion, with or without transcranial exposure through either conventional craniotomy or the subfrontal route. Unlike the endoscopically assisted craniofacial resection, this approach includes actual endoscopic transnasal tumor resection and removal. For non-neoplastic lesions or benign neoplasms, or when the surgeon makes a strategic decision to employ piecemeal removal, tumor removal is done endoscopically. For malignant neoplasms, and when the surgeon decides to avoid piecemeal tumor removal, the endoscopic component of the procedure may be used to explore and free the compartments around the tumor. Using the next-compartment principle, the surgeon dissects at least one compartment away from the tumor. For example, for an esthesioneuroblastoma involving the superior meati and the superior nasal septum, the surgeon may use the endoscopic approach to enter the middle meati on both sides and dissect the ethmoid complex superiorly toward the ethmoid roof. Endoscopic sphenoid sinusotomy may assist in determining the posterior extent of the tumor and can be used to define the posterior resection. Depending on the size and extent of the tumor, it may be removed from above or below the skull base.

Devaiah et al [16] described their modification of anterior craniofacial resection for treatment of esthesioneuroblastoma. They defined their procedures as "endoscopic nasal and anterior craniotomy resection." With this procedure, tumor removal is done both endoscopically and through frontal craniotomy. The procedure begins with piecemeal endoscopic removal of the nasal and sinus components of the tumor. This removal is accomplished with cold instruments, power instrumentation, and unipolar and bipolar cautery. Next, frontal craniotomy is performed, the frontal lobe is elevated off the cribriform plate, and the bony skull base is removed from above by the neurosurgeon. The otolaryngologist assists by placing endoscopes transnasally to determine margins of resection. It should be noted that six of their seven patients received radiation therapy. They reported complete locoregional control in five of the seven patients.

Walch et al [14] described complete endoscopic resection of esthesioneuroblastoma. With their technique, no craniotomy was used. They reported excellent results in three patients. All three patients received stereotactic radiation treatment postoperatively.

Cakmak et al [15] described an endoscopic piecemeal removal of an esthesioneuroblastoma in a pediatric patient. It is not clear if the bony skull base was actually involved in their patient. In fact, they suggested that the tumor may have originated not from the olfactory mucosa in the superior meatus but possibly from the vomeronasal organ, the sphenopalatine ganglion, or the olfactory placode.

Another modification of endoscopic anterior craniofacial resection, which the authors term "the blue sky technique" [9], begins with intracranial exposure through either conventional frontal craniotomy or the subfrontal approach. The anterior cranial fossa floor is explored, and tumor extent and resectability are determined. If dural involvement that requires resection is

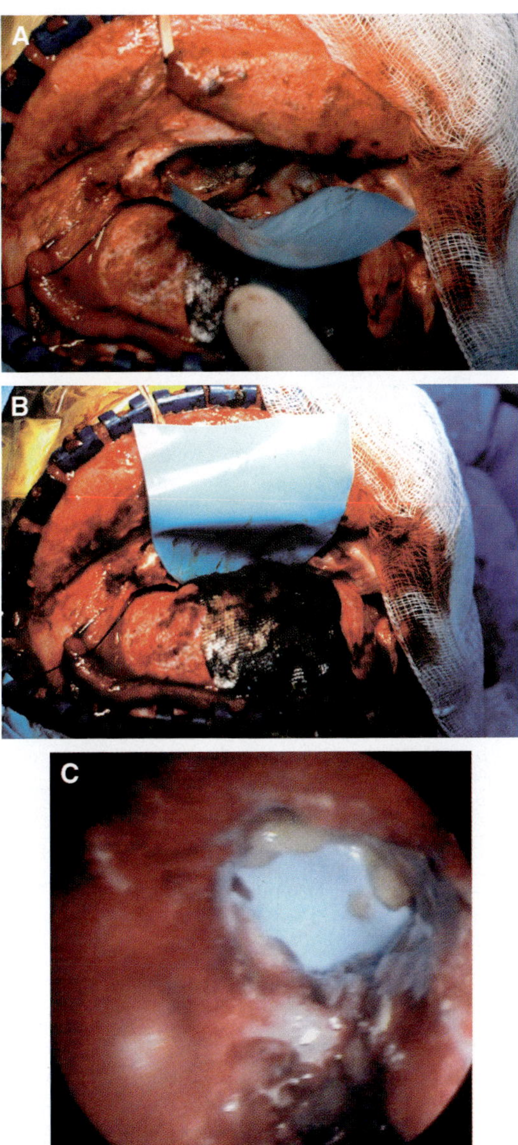

Fig. 5. Endoscopic craniofacial resection–the "blue sky" technique. (*A*) Blue plastic material inserted between the frontal lobe and the anterior skull base. (*B*) Blue material is placed on the anterior skull base lesion. (*C*) "Blue sky" seen endoscopically after removal of the lesion. (*D*) Postoperative coronal CT at the posterior ethmoid region. (*E*) Postoperative coronal CT at the anterior ethmoid region. The left skull base is reconstructed with a pericranial flap (*arrow*). (A and C *from* Har-El G. Anterior craniofacial resection without facial skin incisions. Otolaryngol Head Neck Surg 2004;130:780–7; with permission. B, D, and E *from* Har-El G, Todor R. Endoscopic craniofacial approach for intracranial polyposis–the "blue sky" technique. Skull Base 2003;13:235–9; with permission.)

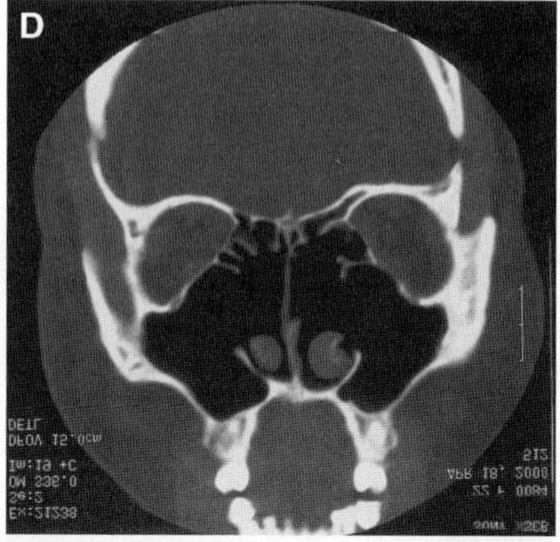

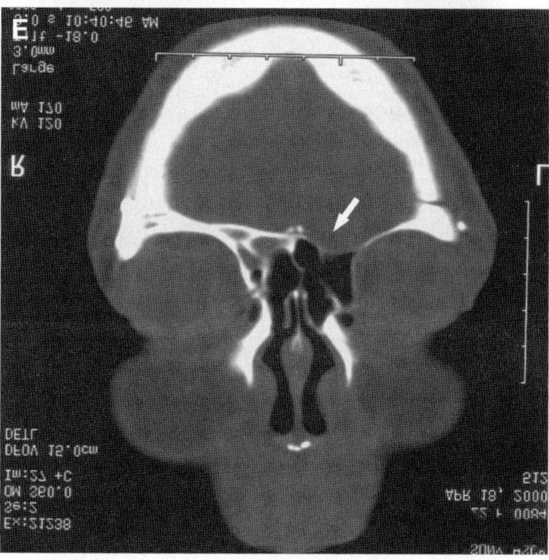

Fig. 5 (*continued*)

identified, it is done at this time. Then, an appropriately sized sheet of colored plastic material, usually a blue plastic surgical cover, is inserted under the dura to rest on the bony skull base covering the entire neoplastic process (Figs. 5A, B). The brain now rests on the blue plastic material, and the bicoronal is scalp flap is temporarily replaced on the cranium. Attention is now directed to the transnasal endoscopic component of the procedure. The blue plastic material provides an excellent visual indication of the location of the skull base. It also prevents accidental dural and brain injury because the surgeon can easily identify it as the superior limit of any surgical manipulation (Fig. 5C). Actual tumor removal is done transnasally with the help of endoscopes. At the end of the procedure, the blue plastic material is removed, and, as in any other form of craniofacial resection, a pericranial or galeal/pericranial flap is developed and transferred to reconstruct the skull base defect (Figs. 5D, E).


## Discussion

Patients and surgeons may be tempted to demand and use the procedures described here for management of sinus and skull base tumors because of their desire to avoid external incision of facial skin. The indications for endoscopic craniofacial resection should be extended with caution. The perceived cosmetic advantages should be weighed against any possibility of compromising the ability to remove tumor completely. It has been repeatedly shown that positive surgical margins at the first extirpative procedure have a negative impact on outcome and overall survival [7].

Additional factors should be considered. A well-placed lateral rhinotomy incision line, with attention to nasal subunits, will have excellent cosmetic results [8]. Therefore, a lateral rhinotomy incision should not be avoided if the use of any other approach may compromise complete tumor removal. In addition, other modifications of ACFR have been described that are based on open, wide exposure without external skin incisions [8]. Examples include the subcranial approach [19], ACFR with the midfacial degloving approach [20–23], and ACFR with LeFort I osteotomy.

The advantages of endoscopic ACFR are not limited to the cosmetic aspect. The use of endoscopes provides better visualization of deeper structures, provides the ability to "look around the corner," and allows the surgeon to avoid the major bony cuts that are used in open procedures for exposure only and not necessarily for tumor removal. For example, transection of the nasolacrimal sac/duct system is usually not required, and postoperative epiphora is avoided. Also, many surgeons challenge the absolute need for en bloc resection and the strict avoidance of piecemeal removal. These issues will certainly make endoscopic ACFR most useful in patients with certain malignancies in certain locations and well-defined extent and in patients with benign or non-neoplastic lesions. For malignancy, the authors have always tried to adhere to the next-compartment rule. Traditionally, it has been their goal, when possible, to perform the first surgical cuts in a space that is at least one compartment away from the tumor. They follow this rule because, within the three-dimensional sinus and anterior skull base complex, margins cannot be defined by centimeters or millimeters the way they are defined for cancer of the tongue, pharynx, and skin. By preoperative examination and imaging studies, the extent of the tumor and the surgeon's ability to remove the entire tumor are assessed. Even if the surgeon decides to use piecemeal removal, complete removal of the tumor should be achieved. If this goal is in doubt, and if the use of an external facial incision will ensure better tumor removal, a classic ACFR should be performed.

## References


[1] Donald PJ. History of skull base surgery. In: Donald PJ, editor. Surgery of the skull base. Philadelphia: Lippinicott-Raven; 1998. p. 3–13.

[2] Dandy WE. Orbital tumor: results following the transcranial operative attack. New York: Oskar Priest; 1941. p. 168–88.

[3] Rae BS, McLean JM. Combined intracranial and orbital operation for retinoblastoma. Arch Ophthalmol 1943;30:437–45.

[4] Smith RR, Klopp CT, Williams JM. Surgical treatment of cancer of the frontal sinus and adjacent areas. Cancer 1954;7:991–4.

[5] Ketcham AS, Wilkins RH, Van Buren JM, et al. A combined intracranial facial approach to the paranasal sinuses. Am J Surg 1963;106:698–703.

[6] Arbit A, Shah JP. Combined craniofacial resection for anterior skull base tumors. Neurosurgical Operative Atlas 1991;1:342–52.

[7] Patel SG, Singh B, Polluri A, et al. Craniofacial surgery for malignant skull base tumors: report of an international collaboration study. Skull Base 2003;13(Suppl 1):7–8.

[8] Har-El G. Anterior craniofacial resection without facial skin incisions. Otolaryngol Head Neck Surg 2004;130:780–7.

[9] Har-El G, Todor R. Endoscopic craniofacial approach for intracranial polyposis–the "blue sky" technique. Skull Base 2003;13:235–9.

[10] Har-El, Todor R. Anterior craniofafacial resection without facial skin incisions. Skull Base 2003;13(Suppl 1):22.

[11] Yuen APW, Fung CT, Hung KN. Endoscopic craniofacial resection of anterior skull base tumor. Am J Otolaryngol 1997;18:431–3.

[12] Thaler ER, Kotapka M, Lanza DC, et al. Endoscopically assisted anterior cranial skull base resection of sinonasal tumors. Am J Rhinol 1999;13:303–10.

[13] Carrau RI, Snyderman CH, Kassam AB, et al. Endoscopic and endoscopic-assisted surgery for juvenile angiofibroma. Laryngoscope 2001;111:483–7.

[14] Walch C, Stammberger H, Anderhuber W, et al. The minimally invasive approach to olfactory neuroblastoma: combined endoscopic and stereotactic treatment. Laryngoscope 2000;110:635–40.

[15] Cakmak D, Ergin NT, Yilmazer C, et al. Endoscopic removal of esthesioneuroblastoma. Int J Pediatr Otorhinolaryngol 2002;64:233–8.

[16] Devaiah AK, Larsen C, Taufik O, et al. Esthesioneuroblastoma: endoscopic nasal and anterior craniotomy resection. Laryngoscope 2003;113:2086–90.

[17] Casiano RR, Numa WA, Falquez AM. Endoscopic resection of esthesioneuroblastoma. Am J Rhinol 2001;15:271–9.

[18] Casiano RR. Anterior skull base resection. In: Endoscopic sinus surgery dissection manual. New York: Marcel Dekker; 2002. p. 99–101.

[19] Raveh J, Laedrach K, Speiser M, et al. The subcranial approach for fronto-orbital and antero-posterior skull base tumors. Arch Otolaryngol Head Neck Surg 1993;119:382–93.

[20] Har-El G, Lucente FE. Midfacial degloving approach to the nose, sinuses and skull base. Am J Rhinol 1996;10:17–22.

[21] Howard DJ, Lund VJ. The role of midfacial degloving in modern rhinologic practice. J Laryngol Otol 1999;113:885–7.

[22] Fliss DM, Zucker G, Amir A, et al. The combined subcranial and midfacial degloving technique for tumor resection: report of three cases. J Oral Maxillofac Surg 2000;58:106–10.

[23] Cocke EW, Robertson JH. Extended unilateral maxillotomy approach. In: Donald PJ, editor. Surgery of the skull base. Philadelphia: Lippincott-Raven; 1998. p. 207–37.

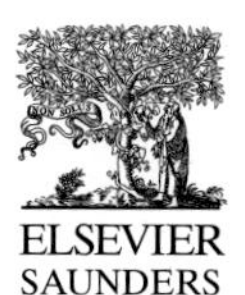

ELSEVIER
SAUNDERS

Otolaryngol Clin N Am
38 (2005) 145–160

OTOLARYNGOLOGIC
CLINICS
OF NORTH AMERICA

# Sentinel Lymph Node Biopsy in Head and Neck Cancer

Ivan H. El-Sayed, MD[a],*,
Mark I. Singer, MD, FACS[a],
Frank Civantos, MD, FACS[b]

[a]*Department of Otolaryngology-Head and Neck Surgery, University of California
Comprehensive Cancer Center, 400 Parnassus Avenue, San Francisco, CA 94143, USA*
[b]*Department of Otolaryngology, University of Miami Hospital and Clinics/Sylvester
Comprehensive Cancer Center, 1475 NW 12 Avenue, Miami, FL 33136, USA*

Sentinel lymph node biopsy (SLNB) is a recently described procedure that has gained a prominent role in the management of early-stage tumors. Currently, the SLNB is routinely used in the management of breast cancer [1], colon cancer [2,3], and cutaneous malignant melanoma (CMM) [4]. It is considered investigational in other solid tumors such as upper gastrointestinal tumors [5], gynecologic cancer [6], penile cancer [7], lung cancer [8], prostate cancer [9], Merkel cell carcinoma [10], and other cancers of the head and neck [11]. For CMM of the head and neck, SLNB provides accurate information regarding the status of the regional nodal basin and provides important prognostic information [12]. In many centers, SLNB is now a standard staging procedure for stage I and II CMM with Breslow thickness greater than 1 mm or other high-risk features [4]. Although no data demonstrate an improved survival for patients undergoing SLNB with CMM, it is widely accepted by patients and the medical community because a negative SLNB can spare 80% of patients a more radical procedure [4].

## History of sentinel node biopsy

The sentinel lymph nodes (SLNs) are the first lymph nodes that receive metastases from the primary tumor. Seaman and Powers [13] described the

* Corresponding author.
*E-mail address:* ielsayed@ohns.ucsf.edu (I.H. El-Sayed).

0030-6665/05/$ - see front matter © 2005 Elsevier Inc. All rights reserved.
doi:10.1016/j.otc.2004.09.004

concept of a first-echelon node. Gould et al [14] labeled this node the "sentinel node" in 1960. In 1977, Cabanas [15] established the basis of the sentinel node theory by demonstrating that a specific node in each groin received lymphatic drainage from primary penile cancer. He concluded tumor cells metastasizing to regional lymphatics would be caught in this node first, and this SLN should be used as a guide to determine the need for lymphadenectomy. Follow-up studies failed to correlate the status of the identified SLN with lymphatic bed, and the SLNB concept was not accepted in the management of penile carcinoma [16,17].

In 1992, Morton et al [18] introduced intraoperative mapping with blue dye as a viable technique to identify the SLN in humans. Using a blue dye injected around the primary tumor, the authors demonstrated they could visually follow the blue-stained lymphatic vessel to the node in 82% of patients. A formal lymphadenectomy was performed to examine the remaining bed for metastases. The identification rate increased significantly with experience for each surgeon. The negative predictive value was close to 98%. This study and subsequent studies found a false-negative rate of less than 5% [18–21].

With blue dye alone, the SLN can be identified in only 80% of patients [18]. Alex and Krag [22] subsequently proposed using lymphoscintigraphy and a handheld gamma probe to identify a SLN. Lymphoscintigraphy alone identifies a SLN in 90% of cases [11]. Recent studies in CMM using the combined techniques of blue dye, preoperative lymphoscintigraphy, and the handheld gamma probe identify a SLN in more than 95% of cases [12,23–27]. These studies indicate the two techniques are complementary because the SLN containing micrometastases may not stain blue but may be radioactive, or it may be blue but not radioactive. Morton et al [28] reviewed data from a multicenter trial and concluded blue dye and radiocolloid with a gamma probe is superior to blue dye alone for detecting CMM. The authors estimated that a surgeon needs 30 consecutive cases to become proficient with this combined technique for CMM. Data from the First International Sentinel Node Biopsy Conference suggest that for oral squamous cell carcinoma, a caseload of 10 is sufficient to identify a SLN in more than 90% of cases [29]. More importantly, when the identified SLN is negative for micrometastases by blue dye staining or radioactivity, the remaining nodal basin is usually negative [4].

Other authors have questioned the importance of using blue dye, particularly for mucosal lesions, where the dye tends to run through the neck quickly, and removal of the primary tumor can help to reduce background activity but delays entry into the neck. Regardless of whether blue dye is used, there is a consensus that the radionuclide represents the more important part of the procedure, with objective numerical ex vivo readings from the lymph node and the surgical bed documenting the presence of a sentinel node [11,25,30–32].

## Sentinel lymph node biopsy in the head and neck

The majority of the melanoma literature concentrates on the extremities and trunk. SLNB in the head and neck presents several unique problems. O'Brien et al [33] describe four difficulties with lymphatic mapping in the head and neck:

1. It is difficult to visualize lymphatic channels using lymphoscintigraphy because of proximity to the injection site.
2. The radiotracer travels fast in the lymphatic vessels.
3. If more than one node is visible, it can be difficult to distinguish first-echelon nodes from second-echelon nodes.
4. The SLN may be small and not easily accessible (eg, in the parotid gland).

Further, the complex drainage patterns of the head and neck have raised concerns that SLNB may not be accurate in the head and neck.

Conflicting data are reported regarding the accuracy of SLNB using the combined technique in the head and neck. Although the sensitivity, often defined as the identification of at least one SLN in a patient, is reported to be around 95% with a low false-negative rate [25,27] Jansen et al [34] reported that a SLN was not identifiable in 10% of head and neck melanomas. The authors concluded that SLNB in the head and neck is technically demanding. Although lymphoscintigraphy alone identifies a SLN in 90% of cases of head and neck melanoma, the gamma camera may not have the resolution needed to distinguish lymphatic vessels and SLNs in close proximity [11]. The gamma probe improves the resolution of nodes in close proximity because the device is held against the tissue during the dissection, and the probe angle is changed. Before skin incision, the gamma probe can resolve a SLN to within 1 cm. The introduction of the handheld gamma probe into one group's practice produced a statistically significant increase in the identification of the SLN from 53% to 92%. Recent studies with large series of patients with melanoma of the head and neck report a SLN identification rate of 75% to 92% with blue dye alone and of more than 96% with combined blue dye and gamma probe detection [24,25,28,32,35–37].

In the head and neck, many factors may affect the accuracy of the SLNB. The definition of sensitivity is evolving because data have revealed multiple channels, and more than one SLN may exist in the head and neck. In the largest study of head and neck melanoma to date, De Wilt et al [36] reported that they identified a SLN in 99% of patients; however, they harvested only 70% of the SLNS identified on preoperative lymphoscintigraphy. O'Brien et al [33] suggest that although one SLN is usually easy to find, it is possible to overlook remaining SLNs. The sensitivity reported for this procedure in many studies should be interpreted cautiously. Another factor identified by de Wilt et al [36] affecting the yield of SLNB is the surgeon's willingness to pursue all the identified channels or SLNs in the parotid region. Further, not all surgeons performing SLNB in the head and neck are specialized head and neck surgeons, and lack of experience may reduce the ability to locate SLNs. Although this point has not been specifically addressed in the literature, it may be one variable affecting the sensitivity reported in large multicenter trials.

There has been no trial of SLNB compared with lymphadenectomy in the head and neck to validate the SLNB technique. Based on the findings of interval nodes, in-transit nodes, and nodes outside of parotid gland region and expected neck regions, it is not clear that a parotidectomy and elective neck dissection would serve as an appropriate control to determine the true accuracy of the SLNB for the head and neck. Clinically, the false-negative rate can be estimated by recurrence in the same lymphatic basin after a negative SLNB. O'Brien et al [33] are frequently cited as finding that disease in the neck recurred in 4 of 16 patients (25%) after a negative SLNB. In this study, SLNs were identified with blue dye and preoperative lymphoscintigraphy without a handheld gamma probe. Chao et al [32] analyzed 2610 patients from the Sunbelt Melanoma Trial database with a median follow-up of 18 months to determine if the rate of recurrence was significantly different than in truncal or extremity melanoma. Although there was some variation in technique used, more than 92% of procedures in each group were performed using radiocolloid. Of the 2610 patients, 321 had primary tumors in the head and neck. There were an average of 1.17, 1.29, and 1.05 nodal basins mapped for head and neck, truncal, and extremity melanomas, respectively. A single nodal basin was harvested in the head and neck in 83% of cases, and more than one was harvested in 17%. On average, 2.8 nodes were harvested in the head and neck, compared with 2.7 in the trunk and 2.1 in the extremities. The same-basin recurrence was 1.9% for the head and neck compared with 0.5% in the extremities and trunk ($P < 0.05$). Other studies report a same-basin recurrence ranging from 0% to 10% [24,26,27,34–36,38,39]. At the University of California at San Francisco, the authors found a 5.6% rate of regional recurrence with a negative SLNB in a review of 80 patients [39]. The follow-up in these studies ranged from 11 to 46 months. Alex [11] reported the longest follow-up to date, with a mean of 6.8 years. Forty-two patients had a SLNB. A positive node was found in five patients. Only one patient without a positive node developed a regional recurrence; in this patient a sentinel node was not located by lymphoscintigraphy and intraoperative mapping with blue dye and gamma probe detection.

With this low false-negative rate, SLNB still seems to be the best staging tool in the head and neck because a SLNB found to be positive for micrometastases is often the only node positive for tumor. The SLN was the only node with metastatic disease in 79% of patients with a positive SLNB undergoing completion lymphadenectomy, and only 1.4% of 72 patients undergoing completion lymphadenectomy had evidence of micrometastases in a non-SLN [12]. Longer follow-up of larger series of patients is needed.

*The rationale and role of sentinel lymph node biopsy in the management of cutaneous malignant melanoma*

Four reasons are cited for performing SLNB in patients with CMM. First, knowledge of the status of the nodal basin provides significant prognostic information for the patient. Second, SLNB identifies patients with regional metastases who may benefit from surgical lymphadenectomy. Third, SLNB identifies patients who are candidates for adjuvant therapy. Fourth, SLNB provides accurate staging information for enrollment in clinical trials [40].

Nodal status is the most important prognostic indicator of patients with CMM, but only 10% to 20% of patients present with occult metastatic nodal disease. Consistent with the expected rate of metastatic disease, a positive SLN is identified in 15% of patients using hematoxylin and eosin stains and SLNB [12]. SLNB is a minimally invasive surgery that can identify patients with occult regional metastases and spare 80% of patients an elective regional lymphadenectomy. Surgical excision is the only proven curative treatment, and elective lymph node dissection (ELND) is recommended for patients with a positive SLNB. The risk of occult regional metastases increases with primary tumor thickness: the risk is 5% for tumors with a thickness of 1 mm, 20% for tumors with thickness of 1 to 4 mm, and 30% to 50% for tumors with a thickness greater than 4 mm [41–43]. Metastatic disease is found on SLNB in 19% of patients with a primary tumor 1.4 to 4 mm thick and in 34% of patients with a primary tumor more than 4 mm thick [12].

No study yet has shown a survival advantage for patients having neck dissection with an N0 neck [33,44], perhaps because 80% of patients undergoing ELND have histologically negative nodes found in the neck specimen, and many patients die of disseminated disease despite having a negative neck [45]. Four prospective clinical trials have failed to demonstrate an advantage of ELND [46–51]. Two of the trials, however, did suggest subgroups may benefit [50,51]. In studies where SLNB was not done, it is possible that the true SLN was outside the surgical area. A SLNB may allow identification and surgical treatment of only those patients with histologically proven nodes [19]. This improved staging will lead to a better assessment of the utility of ELND. Recent data from the World Health Organization trial and the Intergroup Melanoma Surgical trial suggest a significant survival advantage exists for patients with lesions more than 1 mm thick undergoing SLNB compared with patients who have clinically N0 necks staged by clinical examination or ELND [52].

*Sentinel lymph node biopsy provides prognostic information*

Even if the utility of the elective neck dissection is unclear, histologic staging of the regional lymphatics provides important prognostic information for the patient and the physician. For early-stage melanoma, the status of the lymphatic basin is the most important prognostic factor with respect to disease-free and disease-specific survival [12]. In a review of 5346 patients in the American Joint Committee on Cancer (AJCC) database who were clinically N0, the 5-year survival rates were 14% to 30% lower for patients found to have occult regional metastases proven after radical lymphadenectomy or SLNB [53]. The number of nodes involved by tumor is the most important factor associated with survival for stage III disease. Tumor burden within the node is the second most important prognostic indicator. There is a demonstrable survival difference for patients with micrometastases (occult disease detected by SLNB or lymphadenectomy) compared with micrometastases (clinically positive nodes) [37,44,51]. In recognition of its significance, the information provided by SLNB has been incorporated into the staging system in the sixth edition of the AJCC *Cancer Staging Manual* [41], and the AJCC Melanoma Committee recommends all patients with clinical T2 N0 M0, T3 N0 M0, or T4 N0 M0 melanomas have pathologic nodal staging with sentinel lymphadenectomy before entry into clinical trials [53].

*What if micrometastases are identified?*

SLNB identifies patients who may benefit from a completion elective neck dissection and adjuvant therapy including high-dose interferon alpha-2b therapy [54], radiation [55,56], tumor vaccines [57], and immunostimulation [58].

*Is the lymphatic anatomy of the head and neck too complex for sentinel lymph node biopsy?*

Application of the SLNB in the head and neck may be influenced by the complex anatomy. Malignant melanomas of the head and neck are associated with an increased likelihood of recurrence and diminished overall survival compared with other sites [59]. Head and neck CMM of the scalp, face, ear, and neck was traditionally thought to follow standard drainage patterns [60]. Experience with SLNB has revealed unexpected lymphatic drainage patterns in the extremities and the trunk [61–63]. Head and neck lymphatic drainage from the skin is discordant from the traditional expected drainage pathways in 26% to 84%% of cases [38,64–68]. Bilateral or contralateral drainage is reported in 7% to 10% of patients [32,67,68]. Multiple lymphatic channels with multiple SLNs draining from a primary are common [33]. Leong et al [64] found the rate of discordance is greater in the head and neck (48%) than in the lower extremity (5%) or trunk (25%). Unexpected patterns occur mostly with Clark level 5 primaries (13 of 13 patients) in the frontoparietal regions (6 patients) and facial region (7 patients). Other regions of the head and neck are hard to characterize because almost all basins are theoretically possible [38].

Drainage patterns from the skin of the head and neck have led to concern that SLNB may be more difficult in the head and neck [34]. In addition, there are important vital structures at risk of injury. Further, the nodes closest to the primary tumor do not necessarily contain the metastatic disease. Any node receiving direct drainage from the primary tumor is a SLN [33]. A channel could traverse past the upper neck directly to a SLN in the lower neck. In addition, an interval node may occur along the lymphatic vessel before the vessel reaches the expected lymphatic basin, and this node may harbor metastases [69]. Failure to identify and harvest an interval node could lead the surgeon to collect a second-echelon node erroneously. Exploration in the parotid gland or adjacent to vital structures increases the risk of morbidity. Although the lymphatic patterns are complex in the head and neck, this variability argues in favor of a technique that can direct the surgeon and pathologist to the nodes most likely to harbor metastases. A lymph node that occurs outside the predicted lymphatic basin will not be harvested by standard lymphadenectomy without SLNB. The SLNB reduces the number of nodes harvested and allows the pathologist to examine the most important nodes meticulously.

The facial nerve is at risk during SLNB of the head and neck. Nearly one third to one half of head and neck melanomas drain to the periparotid region [32,33,38,70]. Data from the Sunbelt Melanoma Trial, an ongoing multi-institutional study, identified only one temporary facial nerve injury in 95 SLNBs in the parotid region [32]. Fincher et al [38] reported that only 9 of 18 periparotid nodes required a formal facial nerve dissection.

## Science and physiology of lymphoscintigraphy

Lymphoscintigraphy was first described by Sherman and Ter-Pogossian [71]. The earliest lymphoscintigraphy agent used was Gold-198 (Au-198) colloid with a particle size of 5 nm. Greater and earlier uptake was observed with this agent than with any subsequently developed radiocolloids, but it delivered an unacceptably high dose of radiation to the primary site [72]. Other agents studied included Iodine-131 and Technetium-99m (Tc99m), attached to protein or in colloidal form. Tc99m sulfur colloid is advantageous because

1. It emits only gamma rays and has a low overall exposure radiation to the patient and physicians.
2. The half-life of Tc99m is only 6 hours.
3. It has an energy peak of 140 keV, which is within range of most gamma cameras and handheld gamma probes.

The radioisotopes are injected peritumorally and travel into the lymphatics by way of patent junctions through the interstitial space or through the endothelial cells by pinocytosis [73].

The ideal radiotracer would travel quickly to the first-echelon SLNs, where it would be trapped without escaping to the next node. Once in the lymphatic vessels, the particles are filtered through the lymph nodes as they travel to the first-, second-, or third-echelon nodes. Depending on the particle size and the attached molecule, the radioisotopes become trapped in the lymph nodes. The optimal particle size to visualize the maximum number of lymph nodes in a nodal basin is thought to be 5 to 10 nm [72]. Smaller particles are taken up by the vascular capillaries, and larger particles fail to visualize 50% of the normal nodes in the draining basin. The nanocolloid can be used in a filtered or nonfiltered form. The nonfiltered sulfur colloid ranges from 50 to 1000 nm (average 200 nm) [72,74]. The colloid can be filtered to produce a narrower distribution range between 15 and 50 nm [75]. On lymphoscintigraphy, the uptake and distribution of the filtered form is similar to that of antimony sulfur colloid.

Preoperative cutaneous lymphoscintigraphy is performed in the United States with Tc99m-labeled albumin colloid (CIS-US, Inc., Bedford, MA), Tc99m sulfur colloid (CIS-US), or Tc99m human serum albumin (Amersham Mediphysics, Arlington Heights, IL). In Australia, colloidal antimony sulfide is used; human albumin nanocolloid is commonly used in European centers. Approximately 18.5 to 30 mBq (0.5–0.8 mCi) is injected [76]. The variability of tracers used may lead to discordant results among studies [11]. A comparison of colloids in a rabbit model revealed that the highest nodal uptake was 9% for Au-198 followed by 5% for the antimony sulfur colloid. Uptake began immediately and achieved a plateau within 2 hours. The lowest nodal uptake was with sulfur colloid [72]. Clinical experience with CMM has demonstrated that Tc99m sulfur colloid concentrates within the reticuloendothelial system of the regional nodes within 3 to 6 hours [20,77] and can be detected for up to 7 hours without significant leakage. SLNs are frequently identified using lymphoscintigraphy within 1 hour of injection of the radiocolloid and surgically within an additional 3 to 4 hours [77]. An overnight delay is acceptable [78].

## Technique

### Preoperative lymphoscintigraphy

For CMM, an average of 0.5 mCi Tc99m-labeled sulfur colloid is injected intradermally around the primary tumor where it is taken up into the intradermal lymphatics. For the cancers of the upper aerodigestive tract, the best site of injection has not been determined, but typically it is placed in the dermal layer around the lesion and just deep to the lesion. The lymphatic basin is imaged with a gamma camera. The lymphatic channels can be seen within 5 to 10 minutes and imaged for 20 minutes after injection to determine the number of nodal basins and identify which nodes seem to be SLNs.

*Intraoperative mapping*

The patient is taken to the operating room for surgical intraoperative mapping. A gamma probe is used that has a photo-peak at 140 keV with a 10-keV window to optimize detection of Tc99m. The probe's sensitivity is adjusted intraoperatively to the signal intensity by setting the background to zero. The gamma probe can localize a lymph node smaller than 5 mm intraoperatively [79]. The use of a collimator improves resolution of single nodes.

Blue dye, 0.5 mL to 1.0 mL, is then injected intradermally around the primary tumor. Three forms are generally used: methylene blue, isosulfan blue, or patent blue dye. Blue dye stains the SLN for 15 to 45 minutes and may require intraoperative re-injection if it has cleared from the SLN.

Drawbacks of blue dye have been described. Staining of the tissue may obscure tissue planes around the primary tumor. It is difficult to determine the location of the SLN before the skin incision and to verify complete removal of the SLNs using blue dye alone. The surgeon must acquire experience with the procedure to become facile. Further, lymph nodes may be stained for as little as 15 minutes, and re-injection of dye may be necessary [11].

*Intraoperative mapping*

After the blue dye is injected intradermally, lymphatic mapping using a handheld gamma probe is performed. A 2-mm collimator decreases background noise and helps the surgeon locate the node by noting changes in counts in response to changes in the angulation of the probe. The SLN is identified by the skin markings and then with the gamma probe before skin incision. Skin incisions are made over the location of the SLN. In the neck, supraplatysmal flaps are elevated; over the parotid or occipital region, subdermal flaps are elevated. The blue dye–stained lymphatics, if found, are traced to the SLN.

Blue-stained lymphatic vessels are identified and can be traced to the SLN. A gamma probe is often used to identify the SLN by its radioactivity and obviates tracing the blue-stained vessel. There is no threshold amount of radioactivity or blue dye to define a SLN [4]. The highest total radioactive count is measured in the lymphatic basin. After removal of the SLN, the count is remeasured to ensure there are no remaining hot nodes. Remaining nodes that are more than 10% as hot as the hottest node are removed. The 10%-rule is based on findings indicating that 13% of the hottest nodes are not the node with metastatic disease. This recommendation is validated for breast cancer and CMM [30]. Harvested nodes are labeled for the pathologist as SLNs or non-SLNs.

*Risks*

Potential pitfalls of blue dye include a 0.7% to 2% risk of anaphylaxis and extravasation of dye with staining of surgical field, skin tattooing, or delayed wound healing [4,80]. There is a theoretical risk of injury to the facial nerve and other cranial nerves, but the reported incidence is less than 1%. A facial nerve monitor is used, and the facial nerve is identified as appropriate. In the senior author's experience (Dr. Singer), nodes are frequently noted just posterior to the tail of the parotid gland and in the occipital region, areas that do not require identification of the facial nerve. In a series of 80 patients undergoing SLNB in the head and neck at the University of California at San Francisco, only three complications occurred: immediate postoperative hematoma (in 2 patients), and seroma (in 1 patient) [39].

*Pathologic evaluation of the lymph node*

A significant benefit of SLNB is that it identifies for the pathologist the node most likely to harbor metastases. The SLNs are bisected, and each half is cut into multiple sections that are examined using hematoxylin-eosin staining. Negative nodes are further examined using immunohistochemistry staining with HMB-45 and S-100. For squamous cell carcinoma of the head and neck, the use of immunohistochemistry upstages approximately 10% of SLNs, and the use of reverse transcriptase polymerase chain reaction (RT-PCR) technology upstages another 10% [29,81]. Frozen-section analysis for CMM has a poor sensitivity of only 41% [82,83]. Molecular staging using RT-PCR to detect the tyrosinase gene messenger RNA or multiple messenger RNAs has been shown to increase the detection of submicroscopic disease. The significance of detection of the submicroscopic metastases is unknown but is under prospective investigation by the Sunbelt Melanoma Trial [84]. It is hypothesized that the earlier upstaging of these patients may cause a lead-time bias [4] that artificially prolongs their survival. Alternatively, submicroscopic metastases may lack the same pathogenicity as the fully expressed primary tumor. Further study of submicroscopic metastases is necessary to understand their role in the staging and management of patients with CMM.

*Squamous cell cancer of the upper aerodigestive tract*

For squamous cell cancer of the upper aerodigestive tract, most practitioners recommend management of the N0 neck, with either selective neck dissection or radiation, when the risk of occult metastases is 15 to 20%. In the case of oral carcinoma, if SLNB is accurate, formal lymphadenectomy or radiation could be avoided in approximately 70% of patients. Physical examination and imaging studies in the head and neck are currently inadequate to detect the presence of micrometastases. MRI, CT, and ultrasound-guided needle biopsy have a sensitivity of only about 70% in detecting nonpalpable regional disease and a specificity of 100% [85]. Positron emission tomography (PET) has poor sensitivity for tumors less than 5 mm in size [86]. SLNB detects microscopic and submicroscopic disease and seems to correlate well with PET findings [31]. The variability of the lymphatic supply in the upper aerodigestive tract has led to concern about the use of SLNB in the head and neck [87]. Modern anatomic studies demonstrate that the upper aerodigestive tract is not strictly compartmentalized into single segments with a corresponding lymphatic basin; rather, there is frequently bilateral drainage in nearly all areas of the upper aerodigestive tract [88]. A second factor making SLNB difficult is the proximity of the SLN to the primary tumor causing high background noise with the gamma probe and on lymphoscintigraphy.

Alex and Krag [89] performed first successful SLNB for carcinoma of the head and neck in 1996. Pitman et al [90] using blue dye alone were unable to locate a single node and recommended against the procedure. Koch et al [91] had a similarly poor experience using radiocolloid alone. Shoaib et al [92] demonstrated the feasibility of SLNB using radiocolloid with blue dye in a series of patients [92]. In 2000, Alex et al [93] demonstrated accurate localization of SLNs in the head and neck using radiolabeled sulfur colloid and a handheld gamma probe in eight patients with N0 necks and suggested the SLNB has prognostic significance for squamous cell cancer of the upper aerodigestive tract. Several authors have since reported a high identification rate of SLNs in the head and neck. In Europe, in a review of the experience of 22 centers, Ross et al [29] reported an SLN identification rate of 96% for oral squamous cell cancer. For the group of surgeons who had performed fewer than 10 procedures, the identification rate was only 57%. Currently, the American College of Surgeon Oncology Group trial Z0360 is ongoing in an attempt to determine prospectively the accuracy of the radiocolloid SLNB without blue dye for T1/T2 N0 oral squamous cell cancer in comparison to lymph nodes identified in completion neck dissections.

## Other cancers in the head and neck

SLNB has been used in Merkel cell cancer of the skin [11], thyroid carcinoma [94], and skull base lesions. Merkel cell cancer, an aggressive, rare lesion of the skin, frequently metastasizes to the regional lymphatics and distant sites [95]. Treatment of the N0 neck is not well established. SLNB may help direct treatment recommendations in this group of patients.

## Summary

Despite concerns of anatomic complexity, SLNB seems to be safe and effective for CMM in the head and neck. The prognostic information is valuable to the patient and provides a staging tool for the physician. Although the role of neck dissection is controversial, evidence suggests that a subset of patients benefit from ELND. Because the only proven cure for

CMM is surgical resection, identification of subgroups that are amenable to lymphadenectomy may improve their survival. Data provided by SLNB raise questions about the studies on ELND that did not benefit from the information provided by a SLNB.

SLNB has promise for providing important information in other cancers of the head and neck such as Merkel cell cancer or oral squamous cell cancer, but further research is needed.

## References


[1] Giuliano AE, Kirgan DM, Guenther JM, et al. Lymphatic mapping and sentinel lymphadenectomy for breast cancer. Ann Surg 1994;220:391–8 [discussion: 398–401].

[2] Saha S, Nora D, Wong JH, et al. Sentinel lymph node mapping in colorectal cancer–a review. Surg Clin North Am 2000;80:1811–9.

[3] Paramo JC, Summerall J, Poppiti R, et al. Validation of sentinel node mapping in patients with colon cancer. Ann Surg Oncol 2002;9:550–4.

[4] Leong SP. Selective sentinel lymphadenectomy for malignant melanoma. Surg Clin North Am 2003;83:157–85 [vii.].

[5] Kitagawa Y, Fujii H, Mukai M, et al. The role of the sentinel lymph node in gastrointestinal cancer. Surg Clin North Am 2000;80:1799–809.

[6] de Hullu JA, Hollema H, Hoekstra HJ, et al. Vulvar melanoma: is there a role for sentinel lymph node biopsy? Cancer 2002;94:486–91.

[7] Tanis PJ, Lont AP, Meinhardt W, et al. Dynamic sentinel node biopsy for penile cancer: reliability of a staging technique. J Urol 2002;168:76–80.

[8] Liptay MJ, Masters GA, Winchester DJ, et al. Intraoperative radioisotope sentinel lymph node mapping in non-small cell lung cancer. Ann Thorac Surg 2000;70:384–9 [discussion: 389–90].

[9] Wawroschek F, Vogt H, Weckermann D, et al. The sentinel lymph node concept in prostate cancer–first results of gamma probe-guided sentinel lymph node identification. Eur Urol 1999;36:595–600.

[10] Messina JL, Reintgen DS, Cruse CW, et al. Selective lymphadenectomy in patients with Merkel cell (cutaneous neuroendocrine) carcinoma. Ann Surg Oncol 1997;4:389–95.

[11] Alex JC. The application of sentinel node radiolocalization to solid tumors of the head and neck: a 10-year experience. Laryngoscope 2004;114:2–19.

[12] Gershenwald JE, Thompson W, Mansfield PF, et al. Multi-institutional melanoma lymphatic mapping experience: the prognostic value of sentinel lymph node status in 612 stage I or II melanoma patients. J Clin Oncol 1999;17:976–83.

[13] Seaman WB, Powers WE. Studies on the distribution of radioactive colloidal gold in regional lymph nodes containing cancer. Cancer 1955;8:1044–6.

[14] Gould EA, Winship T, Philbin PH, et al. Observations on a "sentinel node" in cancer of the parotid. Cancer 1960;13:77–8.

[15] Cabanas RM. An approach for the treatment of penile carcinoma. Cancer 1977;39:456–66.

[16] Perinetti E, Crane DB, Catalona WJ. Unreliability of sentinel lymph node biopsy for staging penile carcinoma. J Urol 1980;124:734–5.

[17] Wespes E, Simon J, Schulman CC. Cabanas approach: is sentinel node biopsy reliable for staging penile carcinoma? Urology 1986;28:278–9.

[18] Morton DL, Wen DR, Wong JH, et al. Technical details of intraoperative lymphatic mapping for early stage melanoma. Arch Surg 1992;127:392–9.

[19] Thompson JF, McCarthy WH, Bosch CM, et al. Sentinel lymph node status as an indicator of the presence of metastatic melanoma in regional lymph nodes. Melanoma Res 1995;5: 255–60.

[20] Albertini JJ, Cruse CW, Rapaport D, et al. Intraoperative radio-lympho-scintigraphy improves sentinel lymph node identification for patients with melanoma. Ann Surg 1996; 223:217–24.

[21] Uren RF, Howman-Giles R, Thompson JF, et al. Lymphoscintigraphy to identify sentinel lymph nodes in patients with melanoma. Melanoma Res 1994;4:395–9.

[22] Alex JC, Krag DN. Gamma-probe guided localization of lymph nodes. Surg Oncol 1993;2: 137–43.

[23] Kapteijn BA, Nieweg OE, Liem I, et al. Localizing the sentinel node in cutaneous melanoma: gamma probe detection versus blue dye. Ann Surg Oncol 1997;4:156–60.

[24] Bostick P, Essner R, Sarantou T, et al. Intraoperative lymphatic mapping for early-stage melanoma of the head and neck. Am J Surg 1997;174:536–9.

[25] Alex JC, Krag DN, Harlow SP, et al. Localization of regional lymph nodes in melanomas of the head and neck. Arch Otolaryngol Head Neck Surg 1998;124:135–40.

[26] Doting MH, Hoekstra HJ, Plukker JT, et al. Is sentinel node biopsy beneficial in melanoma patients? A report on 200 patients with cutaneous melanoma. Eur J Surg Oncol 2002;28: 673–8.

[27] Wells KE, Rapaport DP, Cruse CW, et al. Sentinel lymph node biopsy in melanoma of the head and neck. Plast Reconstr Surg 1997;100:591–4.

[28] Morton DL, Thompson JF, Essner R, et al. Validation of the accuracy of intraoperative lymphatic mapping and sentinel lymphadenectomy for early-stage melanoma: a multicenter trial. Multicenter Selective Lymphadenectomy Trial Group. Ann Surg 1999;230:453–63 [discussion: 463–5].

[29] Ross GL, Shoaib T, Soutar DS, et al. The First International Conference on Sentinel Node Biopsy in Mucosal Head and Neck Cancer and adoption of a multicenter trial protocol. Ann Surg Oncol 2002;9:406–10.

[30] McMasters KM, Reintgen DS, Ross MI, et al. Sentinel lymph node biopsy for melanoma: how many radioactive nodes should be removed? Ann Surg Oncol 2001;8:192–7.

[31] Civantos FJ, Gomez C, Duque C, et al. Sentinel node biopsy in oral cavity cancer: correlation with PET scan and immunohistochemistry. Head Neck 2003;25:1–9.

[32] Chao C, Wong SL, Edwards MJ, et al. Sentinel lymph node biopsy for head and neck melanomas. Ann Surg Oncol 2003;10:21–6.

[33] O'Brien CJ, Uren RF, Thompson JF, et al. Prediction of potential metastatic sites in cutaneous head and neck melanoma using lymphoscintigraphy. Am J Surg 1995;170:461–6.

[34] Jansen L, Koops HS, Nieweg OE, et al. Sentinel node biopsy for melanoma in the head and neck region. Head Neck 2000;22:27–33.

[35] Schmalbach CE, Nussenbaum B, Rees RS, et al. Reliability of sentinel lymph node mapping with biopsy for head and neck cutaneous melanoma. Arch Otolaryngol Head Neck Surg 2003;129:61–5.

[36] de Wilt JH, Thompson JF, Uren RF, et al. Correlation between preoperative lympho-scintigraphy and metastatic nodal disease sites in 362 patients with cutaneous melanomas of the head and neck. Ann Surg 2004;239:544–52.

[37] Cascinelli N, Belli F, Santinami M, et al. Sentinel lymph node biopsy in cutaneous melanoma: the WHO Melanoma Program experience. Ann Surg Oncol 2000;7:469–74.

[38] Fincher TR, O'Brien JC, McCarty TM, et al. Patterns of drainage and recurrence following sentinel lymph node biopsy for cutaneous melanoma of the head and neck. Arch Otolaryngol Head Neck Surg 2004;130:844–8.

[39] Lin D, Singer MI. 2004. In press.

[40] McMasters KM, Reintgen DS, Ross MI, et al. Sentinel lymph node biopsy for melanoma: controversy despite widespread agreement. J Clin Oncol 2001;19:2851–5.

[41] Balch CM, Buzaid AC, Soong SJ, et al. Final version of the American Joint Committee on Cancer staging system for cutaneous melanoma. J Clin Oncol 2001;19:3635–48.

[42] McMasters KM, Swetter SM. Current management of melanoma: benefits of surgical staging and adjuvant therapy. J Surg Oncol 2003;82:209–16.

[43] Slingluff CL Jr, Stidham KR, Ricci WM, et al. Surgical management of regional lymph nodes in patients with melanoma. Experience with 4682 patients. Ann Surg 1994;219:120–30.

[44] Macripo G, Quaglino P, Caliendo V, et al. Sentinel lymph node dissection in stage I/II melanoma patients: surgical management and clinical follow-up study. Melanoma Res 2004; 14:S9–12.

[45] O'Brien CJ, Petersen-Schaefer K, Ruark D, et al. Radical, modified, and selective neck dissection for cutaneous malignant melanoma. Head Neck 1995;17:232–41.

[46] Sim FH, Taylor WF, Pritchard DJ, et al. Lymphadenectomy in the management of stage I malignant melanoma: a prospective randomized study. Mayo Clin Proc 1986;61:697–705.

[47] Veronesi U, Adamus J, Bandiera DC, et al. Inefficacy of immediate node dissection in stage I melanoma of the limbs. N Engl J Med 1977;297:627–30.

[48] Veronesi U, Adamus J, Bandiera DC, et al. Stage I melanoma of the limbs. Immediate versus delayed node dissection. Tumori 1980;66:373–96.

[49] Veronesi U, Adamus J, Bandiera DC, et al. Delayed regional lymph node dissection in stage I melanoma of the skin of the lower extremities. Cancer 1982;49:2420–30.

[50] Cascinelli N, Morabito A, Santinami M, et al. Immediate or delayed dissection of regional nodes in patients with melanoma of the trunk: a randomised trial. WHO Melanoma Programme. Lancet 1998;351:793–6.

[51] Balch CM, Soong S, Ross MI, et al. Long-term results of a multi-institutional randomized trial comparing prognostic factors and surgical results for intermediate thickness melanomas (1.0 to 4.0 mm). Intergroup Melanoma Surgical Trial. Ann Surg Oncol 2000;7:87–97.

[52] Dessureault S, Soong SJ, Ross MI, et al. Improved staging of node-negative patients with intermediate to thick melanomas (>1 mm) with the use of lymphatic mapping and sentinel lymph node biopsy. Ann Surg Oncol 2001;8:766–70.

[53] Balch CM, Soong SJ, Gershenwald JE, et al. Prognostic factors analysis of 17,600 melanoma patients: validation of the American Joint Committee on Cancer melanoma staging system. J Clin Oncol 2001;19:3622–34.

[54] Kirkwood JM, Strawderman MH, Ernstoff MS, et al. Interferon alfa-2b adjuvant therapy of high-risk resected cutaneous melanoma: the Eastern Cooperative Oncology Group Trial EST 1684. J Clin Oncol 1996;14:7–17.

[55] Stevens G, Thompson JF, Firth I, et al. Locally advanced melanoma: results of post-operative hypofractionated radiation therapy. Cancer 2000;88:88–94.

[56] O'Brien CJ, Petersen-Schaefer K, Stevens GN, et al. Adjuvant radiotherapy following neck dissection and parotidectomy for metastatic malignant melanoma. Head Neck 1997;19: 589–94.

[57] Morton DL, Barth A. Vaccine therapy for malignant melanoma. CA Cancer J Clin 1996;46: 225–44.

[58] Palmer K, Moore J, Everard M, et al. Gene therapy with autologous, interleukin 2-secreting tumor cells in patients with malignant melanoma. Hum Gene Ther 1999;10:1261–8.

[59] Fisher SR, O'Brien CJ. Head and neck melanoma. St. Louis: Quality Medical Publishing; 1998.

[60] Lentsch EJ, Myers JN. Melanoma of the head and neck: current concepts in diagnosis and management. Laryngoscope 2001;111:1209–22.

[61] Uren RF, Howman-Giles R, Thompson JF. Lymphatic drainage from the skin of the back to retroperitoneal and paravertebral lymph nodes in melanoma patients. Ann Surg Oncol 1998; 5:384–7.

[62] Uren RF, Howman-Giles R, Thompson JF, et al. Lymphatic drainage to triangular intermuscular space lymph nodes in melanoma on the back. J Nucl Med 1996;37:964–6.

[63] Uren RF, Howman-Giles RB, Thompson JF, et al. Lymphatic drainage from peri-umbilical skin to internal mammary nodes. Clin Nucl Med 1995;20:254–5.

[64] Leong SP, Achtem TA, Habib FA, et al. Discordancy between clinical predictions vs lymphoscintigraphic and intraoperative mapping of sentinel lymph node drainage of primary melanoma. Arch Dermatol 1999;135:1472–6.

[65] Shah JP, Kraus DH, Dubner S, et al. Patterns of regional lymph node metastases from cutaneous melanomas of the head and neck. Am J Surg 1991;162:320–3.

[66] Wanebo HJ, Harpole D, Teates CD. Radionuclide lymphoscintigraphy with technetium 99m antimony sulfide colloid to identify lymphatic drainage of cutaneous melanoma at ambiguous sites in the head and neck and trunk. Cancer 1985;55:1403–13.

[67] Berman CG, Norman J, Cruse CW, et al. Lymphoscintigraphy in malignant melanoma. Ann Plast Surg 1992;28:29–32.

[68] Morton DL, Wen DR, Foshag LJ, et al. Intraoperative lymphatic mapping and selective cervical lymphadenectomy for early-stage melanomas of the head and neck. J Clin Oncol 1993;11:1751–6.

[69] Uren RF, Howman-Giles R, Thompson JF, et al. Interval nodes: the forgotten sentinel nodes in patients with melanoma. Arch Surg 2000;135:1168–72.

[70] Eicher SA, Clayman GL, Myers JN, et al. A prospective study of intraoperative lymphatic mapping for head and neck cutaneous melanoma. Arch Otolaryngol Head Neck Surg 2002; 128:241–6.

[71] Sherman AI, Ter-Pogossian M. Lymph-node concentration of radioactive colloidal gold following interstitial injection. Cancer 1953;6:1238–40.

[72] Strand SE, Persson BR. Quantitative lymphoscintigraphy I: Basic concepts for optimal uptake of radiocolloids in the parasternal lymph nodes of rabbits. J Nucl Med 1979;20: 1038–46.

[73] Luk SC, Nopajaroonsri C, Simon GT. The architecture of the normal lymph node and hemolymph node. A scanning and transmission electron microscopic study. Lab Invest 1973; 29:258–65.

[74] Frier M, Griffiths P, Ramsey A. The physical and chemical characteristics of sulphur colloids. Eur J Nucl Med 1981;6:255–60.

[75] Hung JC, Wiseman GA, Wahner HW, et al. Filtered technetium-99m-sulfur colloid evaluated for lymphoscintigraphy. J Nucl Med 1995;36:1895–901.

[76] Glass EC, Essner R, Morton DL. Kinetics of three lymphoscintigraphic agents in patients with cutaneous melanoma. J Nucl Med 1998;39:1185–90.

[77] Leong SP, Steinmetz I, Habib FA, et al. Optimal selective sentinel lymph node dissection in primary malignant melanoma. Arch Surg 1997;132:666–72 [discussion: 673].

[78] White DC, Schuler FR, Pruitt SK, et al. Timing of sentinel lymph node mapping after lymphoscintigraphy. Surgery 1999;126:156–61.

[79] Alex JC, Weaver DL, Fairbank JT, et al. Gamma-probe-guided lymph node localization in malignant melanoma. Surg Oncol 1993;2:303–8.

[80] Leong SP, Donegan E, Heffernon W, et al. Adverse reactions to isosulfan blue during selective sentinel lymph node dissection in melanoma. Ann Surg Oncol 2000;7:361–6.

[81] Ross GL, Shoaib T, Scott J, et al. The impact of immunohistochemistry on sentinel node biopsy for primary cutaneous malignant melanoma. Br J Plast Surg 2003;56:153–5.

[82] Tanis PJ, Boom RP, Koops HS, et al. Frozen section investigation of the sentinel node in malignant melanoma and breast cancer. Ann Surg Oncol 2001;8:222–6.

[83] Koopal SA, Tiebosch AT, Albertus Piers D, et al. Frozen section analysis of sentinel lymph nodes in melanoma patients. Cancer 2000;89:1720–5.

[84] Reintgen D, Pendas S, Jakub J, et al. National trials involving lymphatic mapping for melanoma: the Multicenter Selective Lymphadenectomy Trial, the Sunbelt Melanoma Trial, and the Florida Melanoma Trial. Semin Oncol 2004;31:363–73.

[85] Hao SP, Ng SH. Magnetic resonance imaging versus clinical palpation in evaluating cervical metastasis from head and neck cancer. Otolaryngol Head Neck Surg 2000;123:324–7.

[86] Stoeckli SJ, Steinert H, Pfaltz M, Schmid S. Is there a role for positron emission tomography with 18F-fluorodeoxyglucose in the initial staging of nodal negative oral and oropharyngeal squamous cell carcinoma. Head Neck 2002;24:345–9.

[87] Jansen L, Nieweg OE, Peterse JL, et al. Reliability of sentinel lymph node biopsy for staging melanoma. Br J Surg 2000;87:484–9.

[88] Werner JA, Dunne AA, Myers JN. Functional anatomy of the lymphatic drainage system of the upper aerodigestive tract and its role in metastasis of squamous cell carcinoma. Head Neck 2003;25:322–32.

[89] Alex JC, Krag DN. The gamma-probe-guided resection of radiolabeled primary lymph nodes. Surg Oncol Clin N Am 1996;5:33–41.

[90] Pitman KT, Johnson JT, Edington H, et al. Lymphatic mapping with isosulfan blue dye in squamous cell carcinoma of the head and neck. Arch Otolaryngol Head Neck Surg 1998;124: 790–3.

[91] Koch WM, Choti MA, Civelek AC, et al. Gamma probe-directed biopsy of the sentinel node in oral squamous cell carcinoma. Arch Otolaryngol Head Neck Surg 1998;124:455–9.

[92] Shoaib T, Soutar DS, Prosser JE, et al. A suggested method for sentinel node biopsy in squamous cell carcinoma of the head and neck. Head Neck 1999;21:728–33.

[93] Alex JC, Sasaki CT, Krag DN, et al. Sentinel lymph node radiolocalization in head and neck squamous cell carcinoma. Laryngoscope 2000;110:198–203.

[94] Chow TL, Lim BH, Kwok SP. Sentinel lymph node dissection in papillary thyroid carcinoma. ANZ J Surg 2004;74:10–2.

[95] Ott MJ, Tanabe KK, Gadd MA, et al. Multimodality management of Merkel cell carcinoma. Arch Surg 1999;134:388–92 [discussion: 392–3].

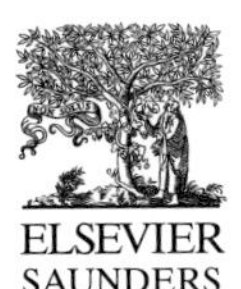

ELSEVIER
SAUNDERS

Otolaryngol Clin N Am
38 (2005) 161–178

OTOLARYNGOLOGIC
CLINICS
OF NORTH AMERICA

# Contemporary Management of Differentiated Thyroid Carcinoma

Richard O. Wein, MD[a],*, Randal S. Weber, MD[b]

[a]Department of Otolaryngology and Communicative Sciences, University of Mississippi Medical Center, 2500 North State Street, Jackson, MS, USA
[b]Department of Otolaryngology-Head and Neck Surgery, University of Texas MD Anderson Cancer Institute, 1515 Holcombe Boulevard, Houston, TX 77030, USA

Well-differentiated thyroid carcinoma remains a relatively uncommon diagnosis with a favorable prognosis. Treatment algorithms continue to evolve with the emergence of new technologies, but the basic surgical approaches to the thyroid have undergone little change.

Thyroid carcinoma currently represents 1.5% of all newly diagnosed cancers in the United States. Approximately 17,000 new cases are diagnosed annually in the United States [1]. This number has increased over the last 25 years from 4.8 to 8.0 cases per 100,000 individuals as of 2001. A female predominance is noted (11.7 female to 4.2 male cases/100,000) with the diagnosis in females nearly doubling during this period. In contrast, the death rate from thyroid carcinoma has remained stable at 0.5 cases per 100,000 individuals [2].

Iodine deficiency is considered to be the most common cause of nodule formation and may be causative in the development of follicular carcinoma. In regions where iodine supplementation has been initiated, rates of follicular cancer have declined, but rates of papillary carcinoma have increased [3].

Investigations into the molecular carcinogenesis of thyroid cancer (eg, into the relationship of the Ret proto-oncogene and the development of papillary carcinoma or the relationship of the Ras signaling pathway and prognosis) are numerous. Future risk analyses may assess the behavior of a specific tumor through the use of biomarker panels and hold the potential for individualizing treatment to specific genetic alterations [4,5].

---

* Corresponding author.
*E-mail address:* rwein@ent.umsmed.edu (R.O. Wein).

## History and physical examination

Several risk factors associated with carcinoma require consideration when evaluating patients with a thyroid mass. An age of less than 15 years or more than 45 years and male sex may immediately place a patient in a higher risk category [6]. Patients with a history of prior radiation exposure are at an increased risk of developing papillary carcinoma. Up to 5% of patients with a history of low-dose radiation exposure develop a thyroid malignancy [7]. When patients present with a solitary thyroid nodule and a history of radiation exposure, 40% of those nodules will harbor a carcinoma [8]. A basic history of coexistent benign thyroid disease such as hyperthyroidism or hypothyroidism should be obtained. Inquiry into a family history of thyroid malignancy and for syndromes such as Cowden's and Gardner's syndromes is also necessary [6]. Ascertaining the presence of symptoms consistent with invasive or compressive growth, such as dyspnea, dysphagia, or dysphonia, is vital.

On physical examination, nodule size of greater than 4 cm should raise concern. Attention should be paid to the relationship of the mass to its surrounding anatomy. Assessment for fixation of the mass, regional adenopathy, recurrent laryngeal nerve paralysis, and piriform or subglottic extension is necessary and may require additional preoperative imaging.

## Evaluation and management of the thyroid nodule

Thyroid nodules are common physical and radiologic findings. Fifty percent of the population has an ultrasound-detectable nodule by age 50 years [9]. The prevalence of nonpalpable nodules of clinical significance (1–1.5 cm in size) in the general population is 2% to 3% [10,11]. Ninety percent of thyroid nodules reflect benign disease such as colloid or adenomatous nodules, follicular adenomas, or lymphocytic thyroiditis. The 10% of nodules that reflect malignant pathology are typically papillary (75%) or follicular (15%) carcinomas.

The initial step in evaluating the routine patient with a thyroid nodule should include a thyroid-stimulating hormone (TSH) level [6]. Ninety-five percent of all nodules are hypofunctional and are considered cold. Assessments that are unnecessary at the initial stage of the evaluation include the routine use of radionuclide scanning, CT or MRI scanning, antithyroid antibodies, or serum levels of T4, T3, or free T3. If the patient's TSH level is normal, the next steps in assessment include obtaining a thyroid ultrasound and performing a fine-needle aspiration (FNA). If a nodule is firm and palpable, FNA can be performed without image guidance. At this stage of the assessment ultrasound examination of the thyroid is beneficial because it offers the ability to assess the number and characteristics of the specific nodules. In patients with solid nonpalpable and cystic nodules, ultrasound-guided FNA offers the best means for obtaining a histologic sample of the nodule of concern. If a patient's TSH level is high, treatment with thyroid hormone replacement should be initiated, and FNA should be performed when the patient is considered euthyroid. Individuals with a low TSH level may have a hyperfunctioning nodule and should be evaluated with a thyroid scan. These lesions have a low likelihood of malignancy.

Ultrasound examination of the thyroid should include an overall assessment of thyroid for size and appearance in addition to a three-dimensional description of the size of specific nodules present. The presence of paratracheal nodes and evidence of invasive qualities of a mass can also be noted on ultrasound examination. Nodules noted on ultrasound examination to be greater than or equal to 1 cm in two dimensions are considered biologically significant. Sixteen percent of patients with palpable nodules will have no nodule detected on ultrasound. The majority of these patients are later diagnosed with Hashimoto's thyroiditis [12,13].

Ultrasound guidance during FNA aids in the biopsy of the cystic nodule because the tissue sampling can focus on the solid component of the nodule. Individuals with multiple nodules on ultrasound evaluation, such as patients diagnosed with multinodular goiter, have the same overall risk of harboring a thyroid carcinoma in another nodule as individuals with a single nodule. Multiple authors examining this issue noted rates of carcinoma in a single nodule ranging from 5% to 17%, whereas rates for multinodular patients ranged from 5% to 13% [14–16]. Approximately 15% of individuals with multinodular goiter and a palpable solitary nodule have a second non-palpable nodule that is greater than 1 cm in size [12,13].

The results of a thyroid nodule FNA should yield only a limited number of potential interpretations, such as benign goiter, malignancy, follicular neoplasm, or nondiagnostic sample. A diagnosis of benign goiter can reflect the presence of a nodular goiter or lymphocytic thyroiditis. The FNA result of follicular neoplasm should be viewed as an indeterminate finding because it may reflect benign or malignant disease. A nondiagnostic FNA may be described as demonstrating findings consistent with cyst contents or rare/scant/scattered/insufficient follicular cells for diagnosis. FNA of thyroid nodules has a reported sensitivity greater than 92% with a specificity of about 91% to 97.5% [17,18]. The positive predictive value for FNA may be compromised by the follicular indeterminate result that occurs.

For individuals with benign cytology on FNA, no therapy is required. The thyroid ultrasound allows documentation of the size of the nodule and the sonographic appearance of the thyroid gland for later comparison. Individuals should be re-examined for a change in the nodule size in 6 to 9 months. If the nodule is the same size or smaller by ultrasound, the patient should continue to be followed for re-examination on a yearly basis. If the nodule has increased in size, a repeat FNA should be performed.

When patients undergo serial ultrasounds, it is necessary to define what constitutes growth on the repeat examination. An increase of more than 15% in the size of a nodule in two dimensions is an accepted parameter for defining enlargement, but others choose to follow overall volume change. When serial FNA is performed, the repeat FNA should be performed approximately 3 months later. In one study, when patients underwent repeat FNA on the same nodule for a result previously classified as "non-diagnostic" or "indeterminate for neoplasm," the risk of malignancy on future evaluations was 49% [19].

The indications for obtaining a thyroid scan include individuals who have follicular cytology on FNA. Euthyroid patients with a hyperfunctioning nodule do not require surgery. Nodules that are hyperfunctional tend to be TSH-independent and unresponsive to levothyroxine when attempts are made to suppress the nodule. Cold nodules requiring biopsy may appear in patients with suppressed TSH (eg, in patients with Grave's disease).

Regardless of findings on ultrasound examination, there are clinical presentations that are highly suggestive of underlying malignancy. Hamming et al [20] noted a 71% risk of malignancy in patients presenting with the clinical findings of rapid tumor growth, hard nodules, fixation to adjacent structures, vocal cord paralysis, and enlarged regional lymph nodes. The presence of microcalcifications on ultrasound examination is also suggestive of papillary carcinoma. Chan et al [21] reported a 42% incidence of microcalcifications in patients with known papillary carcinomas. The sensitivity, specificity, and accuracy of microcalcifications for indicating the presence of papillary carcinoma on ultrasound examination are 36%, 93%, and 76%, respectively [22].

## Treatment considerations—pathology

Papillary and follicular carcinomas represent approximately 85% of all thyroid cancers, with papillary carcinomas comprising the majority [23].

When a diagnosis of follicular neoplasm is obtained on FNA, 80% of the nodules represent benign disease, and the remaining 20% represent a thyroid carcinoma. Of this 20%, up to 50% have the diagnosis of a follicular variant of papillary carcinoma. For patients with follicular carcinoma the most important prognostic parameter is age, not sex. Patients 45 years of age or older at the time of diagnosis have a worse prognosis than their younger counterparts. Individuals with carcinomas greater than 5 cm fare worse, probably because of extracapsular spread. Patients with vascular invasion do worse than individuals with capsule invasion. Insular carcinoma is also considered to be a variant of follicular carcinoma that presents with more advanced-stage disease at diagnosis, a higher frequency of metastasis, and a decreased survival when compared with pure follicular carcinoma [24].

Papillary carcinoma has a number of variants requiring special consideration. The diffuse sclerosing variant is a rare subtype that tends to present in women younger than 25 years of age. Tumor size is large at presentation (mean, 6.9 cm) with 100% of patients developing regional lymph node metastases. Despite these factors, prognosis seems to be favorable when aggressive care is rendered [25]. The tall cell variant, representing approximately 5% of papillary carcinomas, is also considered an aggressive subtype with a worse prognosis. Typical presentation is in the older patient with a large tumor, extrathyroidal extension, and nodal metastases [26]. The follicular variant of papillary carcinoma, representing approximately 24% of cases, is more frequently multicentric but has clinical behavior similar to pure papillary carcinoma [27]. When a preoperative FNA returns the diagnosis of papillary carcinoma, the accuracy of the FNA diagnosis approaches 100% and does not require intraoperative frozen-section confirmation.

Hürthle cell carcinomas, considered by some to be a variant of follicular carcinomas, represent only 3% of all thyroid tumors. Ipsilateral lymph node metastases are present in 25% of patients [28]. In a review of 127 patients diagnosed with a Hürthle cell neoplasm, 70% were noted to have carcinomas. Forty percent of these patients eventually died from thyroid carcinoma. In patients with metastases, only 38% of lesions demonstrated uptake of radioactive iodine (RAI) [29].

The term "microcarcinoma" is used to refer to lesions that less than 1 cm in size in patients without evidence of lymph node metastases. Most authors consider these lesions to be incidental and to be adequately treated when removed by lobectomy [1,30].

**Preoperative evaluation**

For individuals with symptoms suggestive of a potentially invasive carcinoma, such as dysphonia, dysphagia, or stridor, assessment beyond the routine physical examination is necessary. Flexible laryngoscopy is crucial preoperatively for identifying patients with vocal cord paralysis suggestive of recurrent laryngeal nerve invasion or laryngeal infiltration. Piriform asymmetry, intraluminal masses, and pooling of secretions suggestive of aerodigestive tract dysfunction should prompt additional radiologic evaluation. MRI allows excellent soft tissue evaluation for findings such as cervical esophageal invasion with the use of a contrast material that will not conflict with potential future treatments. CT scan, although a readily accessible imaging option, requires the administration of an iodinated contrast agent that can delay the use of RAI postoperatively for 4 to 6 weeks. In selected patients panendoscopy before surgical resection allows assessment of intraluminal spread of tumor and aids in surgical planning and developing a reconstructive strategy.

**Staging**

The staging for thyroid cancer, as defined by the American Joint Committee on Cancer (AJCC), recently underwent minor changes in the sixth edition of the AJCC *Cancer Staging Manual* [31]. The current method is based upon the primary tumor (T), regional lymph node (N), and distant metastasis staging (M). The TNM classification and stage grouping for papillary and follicular carcinoma are shown in Box 1. When staging is performed for patients with multifocal tumors, the largest nodule is used for the purposes of primary tumor staging. Combined clinical (preoperative) and pathologic (postoperative) staging is necessary for the purposes of establishing a reference point for future care and for the statistical entry of patients into cancer registries.

## Operative treatment

Because differentiated thyroid carcinoma is biologically less aggressive than other histologies encountered in the head and neck, the surgical approach differs in several ways from the local and regional management of squamous cell carcinoma of the head and neck. Surgical therapy for the majority of well-differentiated thyroid carcinomas should be tailored to the eradication of macroscopic disease while preserving the patient's capacity for functional speech and swallowing and parathyroid preservation. For patients considered at high risk, little debate exists that total thyroidectomy is the procedure of choice. Controversy over the extent of thyroid surgery in low-risk patients (ie, lobectomy [6,32–34] versus total thyroidectomy [26,35,36]) is well documented within the literature and is based on retrospective data analysis. A randomized, prospective trial comparing lobectomy versus total thyroidectomy in the low-risk patient has not been performed. Such a study is impractical given the long follow-up necessary to detect a difference in survival or local failure. The favorable long-term prognosis for most patients with well-differentiated carcinoma drives this debate. The benefits offered in local control and survival with the use of postoperative RAI and thyroid hormone suppression are compelling evidence favoring total thyroidectomy (for tumors > 1.5 cm) to give patients access to these adjunctive therapies [37,38]. Several factors, including performance of risk analysis, can also guide the surgeon in selecting the surgical treatment that is best for the individual patient. Commonly used methods of risk analysis include the AGES (*age, grade, extent, size*) [32], AMES (*age, metastases* [distant], *extent, size*) [39], and MACIS (*metastasis*, patient *age, completeness* of resection, local *invasion*, and tumor *size*) [40] assessments. Finally, the expectations and philosophy of the endocrinologist participating in the care of the patient may significantly affect the type of procedure selected [41].

Use of intraoperative frozen-section histopathologic examination of tissue is also a controversial topic. Its use is reasonable in the patient with the cytologic diagnosis of follicular neoplasm or findings suspicious for papillary carcinoma but not diagnostic for carcinoma. In this scenario, provided that the surgeon and the pathologist have a good working relationship and the capability to establish a more definitive diagnosis,

**Box 1. TNM staging for papillary and follicular carcinoma [31]**

*Primary tumor (T)*
TX Primary tumor cannot be assessed
T0 No evidence of primary tumor
T1 Tumor 2 cm or less in greatest diameter, limited to the thyroid
T2 Tumor > 2 cm and < 4 cm in greatest diameter, limited to the thyroid
T3  Tumor > 4 cm in greatest diameter and limited to the thyroid or any tumor with minimal extrathyroidal extension (eg, extension to sternothyroid muscle or perithyroidal soft tissues)
T4a Tumor of any size extending outside the thyroid capsule to invade subcutaneous soft tissues, larynx, trachea, esophagus, or recurrent laryngeal nerve
T4b Tumor invading prevertebral fascia or encases carotid artery or mediastinal vessels

*Regional lymph nodes (N)*
NX Regional nodes cannot be assessed
N0 No regional lymph node metastases
N1 Regional lymph node metastases
N1a Metastasis to level VI (pretracheal, paratracheal, and prelaryngeal nodes)
N1b Metastasis to unilateral, bilateral, or contralateral cervical or superior mediastinal lymph nodes

*Distant metastasis (M)*
MX Distant metastasis cannot be assessed
M0 No distant metastasis
M1 Distant metastasis

*Stage grouping (for papillary and follicular carcinoma)*
Under 45 years of age
   Stage I Any T Any N Any M
   Stage II Any T Any N M1
45 years of age and older
   Stage I T1 N0 M0
   Stage II T2 N0 M0
   Stage III T3 N0 M0
         T1 N1a M0
         T2 N1a M0
         T3 N1a M0
   Stage IVa T4a N0 M0
         T4a N1a M0
         T1 N1b M0
         T2 N1b M0
         T3 N1b M0
         T4a N1b M0
   Stage IVb T4b Any N M0
   Stage IVc Any T Any N M1

frozen-section examination can spare a patient from a second completion thyroidectomy surgery. Given the need to establish capsular or vascular invasion to confirm the diagnosis of carcinoma, individuals with the pre-operative diagnosis of follicular neoplasm are more likely to require a completion procedure if the diagnosis of follicular carcinoma is rendered on permanent histopathologic evaluation of the initial specimen [42].

Although the operative technique for thyroidectomy is well described, the importance of identifying and dissecting the recurrent laryngeal nerve in addition to preserving and, when necessary, re-implanting the parathyroid gland cannot be overemphasized. A comprehensive understanding of the anatomic relationships of this region and their variants is necessary for successful primary and re-operative approaches.

Electromyography has been used to monitor the recurrent laryngeal nerve in selected settings. For patients undergoing a second procedure in a previously operated bed (eg, paratracheal node dissection after total thyroidectomy), the laryngeal electromyogram can be helpful. Electrodes mounted within an endotracheal tube or placed within the thyroarytenoid muscle after intubation can indicate to the surgeon when dissection extends to the proximity of the recurrent laryngeal nerve and potentially prevent injury when operating in a scarred bed of tissue [43]. The role of electromyography in primary surgery is unclear, and its use will probably not lessen the risk for nerve injury.

In the setting of a FNA indeterminate for malignancy, such as with follicular neoplasm, one of four potential philosophies may be adopted. A wait-and-watch approach may be appropriate for selected patients with significant coexisting medical conditions that make them poor operative candidates. Serial ultrasound to determine growth and repeat FNA may be used to support further the need for treatment. Thyroid lobectomy can be performed with the plan to allow the final histopathologic interpretation to determine whether a completion thyroidectomy is required. This approach offers the patient the possibility of a smaller procedure than a total thyroidectomy with a lower risk for complications and might avoid the need for lifelong thyroid hormone supplementation. When a follicular neoplasm represents a follicular variant of papillary carcinoma, frozen-section examination may provide the intraoperative diagnosis of malignancy, allowing immediate completion thyroidectomy and thereby sparing the need for a second procedure and hospitalization. Frozen-section diagnosis is not always accurate, and false positives do occur. An experienced pathologist is required to avoid error in diagnosis. Finally, the plan for a single operative procedure (ie, total thyroidectomy), regardless of benign or malignant final histopathologic diagnosis, may appeal to some patients who wish to have only one procedure and who are willing to take lifelong thyroid supplementation, provided the surgery can be performed with very low surgical morbidity. Subtotal thyroidectomy is rarely indicated in the treatment of the patient with thyroid carcinoma.

For individuals undergoing unilateral surgery with the potential need for future completion thyroidectomy, the strap muscles overlying the remaining lobe should be left undisturbed to preserve the fascial plane for future dissection. In a series of patients undergoing completion thyroidectomy, 47% of patients with papillary carcinoma and 33% with follicular carcinoma had one or more foci of carcinoma in the remaining lobe [44]. Pasieka et al [45] obtained similar numbers in their review and noted that the presence of multifocal disease in the initial lobectomy specimen was associated with a higher likelihood of cancer in the remaining lobe. Although an increased risk of complications is a concern with completion thyroidectomy, Kupferman et al [46] reported a 13.9% rate of transient postoperative hypocalcemia and no episodes of recurrent laryngeal nerve paralysis in their series of 36 patients.

*Invasive carcinoma*

The locally invasive presentation of well-differentiated thyroid carcinoma occurs in less than 5% of all cases. The most common pathology involved is papillary carcinoma. There is a male predominance with patients presenting at a higher mean age than those with noninvasive disease [47]. Invasive thyroid carcinoma spreads by direct extension from the primary tumor or from extracapsular spread of paratracheal nodal metastasis. Tumor at the primary site has the capacity for invasion through the cricothyroid membrane or the thyroid cartilage anteriorly or may extend posteriorly to wrap around the thyroid cartilage and present in the region of the piriform sinus. Extracapsular spread from paratracheal nodes tends to invade laterally in the region of the tracheoesophageal groove [48]. McCaffrey et al [47], in reviewing the 50-year experience at the Mayo Clinic, reported on 262 patients with invasive thyroid carcinoma. The sites of invasive presentation were trachea (37%), esophagus (21%), recurrent laryngeal nerve (47%), strap musculature (53%), larynx (12%), and other structures (30%). Patients who present with regional metastases (41%) are more likely to have extrathyroidal extension [49].

The goals of treatment for invasive thyroid carcinoma include prevention of hemorrhage and airway obstruction, preservation of a functional upper aerodigestive tract, prevention of locoregional recurrence, and long-term survival. Frequently the mandate for removing all gross disease is at odds with function-sparing surgery. Several authors have advocated a conservative approach of shaving the tumor [47,48,50,51] off the tracheal wall, but other authors advocate more aggressive approaches to accomplish a complete removal of tumor [52,53]. Few disagree that the goal in treating invasive thyroid carcinoma is to remove all macroscopic disease noted at the time of surgery. The controversy lies in the degree of resection required to accomplish this result. For individuals with limited tracheal deficits but gross intraluminal spread of tumor, window and sleeve resections are necessary. For larger defects, up to one third the circumference of the tracheal, use of sternocleidomastoid and pectoralis major myoperiosteal flaps over T-tubes has been described [54]. For larger defects, tracheal resection with re-anastomosis with release procedures while preserving at least one recurrent laryngeal nerve has been described with favorable results [55]. McCaffrey et al [47] retrospectively compared three groups of patients undergoing surgery for thyroid carcinoma with limited tracheal invasion. These groups included individuals undergoing complete surgical excision (group I), shave resection with the potential for microscopic residual disease (group II), and incomplete resection with macroscopic residual disease remaining (group III). The overall 5-year survival was 79%. No significant difference was noted in survival between groups I and II, whereas survival in group III was the lowest. The authors concluded that for selected patients shave resection is a viable option that allows preservation of upper aerodigestive tract anatomy without compromising survival. The importance of postoperative RAI therapy and possible external beam radiation were also stressed.

Esophageal invasion, when present, tends to invade only the outer muscular layers of the esophagus. Because achieving wide tumor-free margins is less of an issue with thyroid carcinoma than with squamous cell carcinoma, limited resection without intraluminal entry is possible. When limited intraluminal invasion is encountered, primary closure of the defect after resection is an option when closure does not predispose to stricture formation. When extensive resections of the esophagus are required, options for reconstruction with pedicled and free tissue transfer parallel those described in the literature for the treatment of squamous cell carcinoma [56].

When a patient presents for thyroidectomy and the preoperative examination indicates paralysis of the recurrent laryngeal nerve, attempts to save the nerve at the time of surgery should not be pursued. Primary thyroplasty may be considered in this scenario. When the recurrent laryngeal nerve is noted to be functional preoperatively, attempts should be made to preserve the nerve if possible. Falk and McCaffrey [57] retrospectively compared patients who had a functional recurrent laryngeal nerve sacrificed at the time of thyroidectomy with those with nerve preservation and noted that complete resection of tumor and nerve sacrifice offered no survival benefit over potentially incomplete resection of tumor and nerve preservation.

Laryngeal invasion requires the surgeon to be aware of the various options in conservation laryngeal surgery if the goal of avoiding total laryngectomy is possible. Vertical partial laryngectomy may be appropriate for patients with unilateral disease, whereas a supracricoid partial laryngectomy may be considered for extensive anterior invasion [56]. The indications for total laryngectomy include extensive laryngeal spread beyond the scope of organ-preservation surgery and involvement of more than one third of the cricoid ring [48].

*Regional metastasis*

Subcapsular lymphatic vessels drain the intraglandular lymphatics. Cross-communication of lymphatics may occur with the contralateral lobe and isthmus. Lymphatic channels parallel venous drainage. First-echelon nodal drainage is to the paralaryngeal, paratracheal, and the prelaryngeal (Delphian) nodes generally considered to be level VI. The second level of drainage includes the upper, mid, and lower jugular nodal groups (levels II, III, and IV) in addition to the inferior spinal accessory nodes (level V). Bilateral spread is common. Regional spread to levels Ia and Ib (submental and submandibular nodal groups) is uncommon. Upper mediastinal and retropharyngeal lymph node metastasis may also occur in selected lesions.

Occult nodal metastases may occur in up to 90% of cases [58]. Bilateral spread is seen in 30% of cases. Mediastinal spread may occur in about 15% of patients. Level I spread accounts for fewer than 5% of nodal metastases. Regional metastases may also occur in patients with no detectable primary thyroid lesion. Although elective neck dissection in the setting of papillary carcinoma will detect occult spread in approximately 50% of patients [59], the performance of the neck dissection is reported to have no impact on survival [60]. Although the impact of regional metastases in younger patients seems to be minimal, clinically apparent regional metastases do correlate with a poorer overall survival and the risk for recurrence in patients over 45 years of age and older [61,62].

Radiologic imaging for regional spread of carcinoma includes ultrasonography, CT, and MRI. Ultrasound may allow detection of occult nodal disease and is most accurate when combined with FNA. Serial ultrasound examinations can be used to assess changes in nodal size. Diagnostic imaging criteria for CT or MRI include recurrent disease, clinical lymph node metastases, vocal cord paralysis, fixation of the tumor mass to adjacent anatomy, and the presence upper aerodigestive of symptoms suggestive of invasive disease. Imaging characteristics that may be consistent with nodal metastases include a solid, calcified, cystic, or hemorrhagic appearance. On MRI, colloid has high signal intensity on T1-weighted images and when detected within the substance of a lymph node is suggestive of regional metastasis. Imaging is helpful in detecting the location and extent of metastases.

The type of neck dissection is dictated by the extent of disease. Routine performance of radical and modified radical neck dissections is not necessary in the setting of limited, well-defined regional disease. Functional (level II–V) and selective (anterolateral level II–IV) neck dissections allow the removal of macroscopic disease while minimizing the risk of associated complications.

Paratracheal nodal dissection in the setting of thyroid carcinoma has been well described in the literature [63]. At the time of thyroidectomy, the paratracheal region should be examined and dissected if clinically positive nodes are encountered. During the procedure the recurrent laryngeal nerve should be located inferiorly and dissected superiorly. Additionally, the superior parathyroids should be avoided given that the lymph nodes of the central neck lie below the level of the inferior thyroid artery. Dissection should extend to the anterior-superior mediastinum and should allow examination posteriorly to the retroesophageal region. In one series, complications such as transient paralysis of the recurrent laryngeal nerve and transient hypoparathyroidism were seen in 13% and 21% of patients, respectively, who underwent central compartment dissection with thyroidectomy and lateral neck dissection. No cases of permanent hypoparathyroidism were experienced [64]. Strategies to avoid these complications in patients requiring re-operation include MRI- and ultrasound-guided FNA to localize the disease and intraoperative monitoring of the recurrent laryngeal nerve.

## Postoperative treatment and follow-up

The treatment algorithms for the postoperative care and long-term follow-up of patients with thyroid carcinoma are undergoing modification with the introduction of recombinant human TSH (rhTSH). Standard regimens have relied on thyroid hormone withdrawal after total thyroidectomy. Patients discharged after surgery were given triiodothyronine (T3), which does not suppress TSH, for approximately 3 weeks. Approximately 2 weeks before RAI whole-body scan (WBS), T3 supplementation was discontinued while the patient remained on a low-iodine diet. If a patient's TSH level had climbed to greater than 25 mU/L, the RAI WBS (using approximately 2 mCi) was performed [1]. After total thyroidectomy, residual thyroid tissue is often noted on the RAI WBS. After adequate surgery, uptake in the thyroid bed should be less than 3%.

Studies have demonstrated the usefulness of postoperative RAI in decreasing the local recurrence and mortality rates in patients with stage II and stage III well-differentiated thyroid carcinoma. For this reason, the routine use of postoperative RAI and thyroid hormone suppression has been advocated for patients with primary tumors larger than 1.5 cm [37,38].

RAI administration can have complications that include radiation thyroiditis (when a large remnant is present), dysphagia, sialoadenitis, glossodynia, tumor edema and hemorrhage, injury to reproductive organs, pulmonary fibrosis (in the setting of extensive lung metastases), and leukemia.

Recent developments, most notably the increasing clinical experience with rhTSH, have led to protocols that now allow patients at low risk for persistent or recurrent disease to be discharged on T4 (levothyroxine) after total thyroidectomy. The patient receives rhTSH weeks later in preparation for radioactive iodine uptake WBS [65]. Based on the results of the WBS, therapeutic RAI can then be administered for the presence of persistent local, regional, or distant disease. The rhTSH allows the quicker clearance of RAI with the potential for fewer side effects and as a result may allow an increase in the dose of RAI administered to patients [66]. Additionally, patients no longer need to experience symptoms of prolonged hypothyroidism before WBS.

Haugen et al [67] demonstrated that when a combination of RAI WBS and serum thyroglobulin (Tg) was performed after rhTSH stimulation, the assays together detected the remnant thyroid tissue or cancer within the thyroid bed in 93% of patients and in 100% of patients with metastatic disease.

Mazzaferri et al [68] reviewed the false-negative rate of surveillance studies in patients with distant metastases and low baseline serum Tg levels (less than 1 µg/L) during TSH suppression therapy. The article compared WBS after thyroid hormone withdrawal or rhTSH with Tg levels after rhTSH stimulation. WBS detected only 19% of the cases with metastases. In comparison, rhTSH-stimulated Tg levels (Tg > 2 µg) can identify the presence of persistent disease in approximately 90% of patients harboring recurrence or metastasis. Based on the results of this review of 10 studies comprising approximately 1600 patients examining the issue of monitoring in the low-risk patient, the authors concluded that assessment of the TSH-stimulated (with either rhTSH or thyroid hormone withdrawal) assessment was sensitive enough to be used alone, without WBS, to monitor patients long-term.

Patients who are found to have elevated rhTSH-stimulated Tg levels (>2 µg/L) and negative RAI WBS are evaluated with positron emission tomography (PET) imaging [68,69]. Patients who are PET positive and RAI WBS negative have a poor prognosis [70] and are not candidates for therapeutic RAI [71]. Patients with tumors that fail to take up iodine have more aggressive pathologies such as insular, Hürthle cell, or anaplastic carcinomas [72–74]. In this setting, CT scan and MRI may be warranted to establish if the patient is a surgical candidate. Using external beam radiation may also be reasonable.

In a consensus report defining the role of serum Tg in the monitoring of low-risk thyroid carcinoma patients, Mazzaferri et al [68] suggested a surveillance algorithm based on the results of multiple studies. When patients are considered clinically disease free for 6 months to 1 year after surgery and RAI therapy, Tg levels are followed while the patient is on thyroid hormone replacement therapy. When Tg is detectable, neck ultrasound and chest radiographs are advised, and RAI therapy or surgery is considered. A WBS is obtained in the posttreatment period to assess remaining disease.

In patients with undetectable Tg levels, rhTSH-stimulated Tg levels are assessed 72 hours after administration. In patients with Tg levels greater than 2 µg/L, an approach similar to that taken for patients with unstimulated detectable Tg is taken to assess for the location of recurrent disease. In patients with elevated Tg levels and a negative WBS, a fluoro-deoxyglucose PET scan is performed in an attempt to isolate the recurrent disease and consider the options for treatment. For patients in whom the rhTSH-stimulated Tg is between 0.6 and 2 µg/L, obtaining a yearly rhTSH-stimulated Tg level is advocated to assess spontaneous decline in Tg levels or a rise indicating the presence of recurrent disease. In individuals with a stimulated Tg level less than 0.6 µg/L, an annual Tg level is advocated during TSH suppression.

Although not a first-line therapy, external beam radiation may have a role in the treatment in patients with non–RIA-avid tumors and invasive or recurrent thyroid carcinoma, gross residual tumor, or unresectable disease. In patients older than 45 years of age with minimal microscopic residual disease or extrathyroidal extension, external beam radiation has shown evidence of decreasing local recurrence [75].

## Distant metastases

The treatment of distant metastases relies predominantly on RAI and external beam radiation. Guidelines from the National Comprehensive Cancer Network categorize treatment options based on the site of metastasis. For solitary central nervous system metastases options include neurosurgical consultation, external beam radiation, and RAI treatment in RAI-avid tumors after treatment with rhTSH. Steroid prophylaxis is used given the potential for tumor edema with rhTSH administration. For bone metastases options include surgical palliation, external beam radiation, RAI treatment in RAI-avid tumors, and bisphosphonate therapy. For metastases to extracervical sites, options include selective surgical resection in symptomatic patients, RAI, external beam radiation, and systemic chemotherapy [6]. The value of metastasectomy was confirmed in a review of the National Institutes of Health experience by Pak et al [76]. In 29 patients with nonmedullary thyroid carcinoma, 47 surgeries were performed for distant metastasis at various sites. Cumulative 5- and 10-year survival rates in the series were 78.5% (+/−8.4%) and 50.2% (+/−12.5%), respectively. Patients with distant metastases who are under 45 years of age, have metastases to only bone or lung, and were treated with RAI fared the best in terms of disease-specific survival [77].

## Prognosis

In addition to the standard TNM system, a number of systems have been developed to gauge risk-group classification. The classifications focus on parameters that are well established in the literature as risk factors for a poorer prognosis. A parameter common to all scoring systems is age given that patients over 45 years of age have a worse outcome than their younger counterparts. Larger primary tumor size and extension and the presence of metastases increase a patient's stage and affect 5-year survival. For papillary carcinoma the 5-year relative survival rates by stage are 100% for stages I and II, 95.8% for stage III, and 45.3% for stage IV. For follicular carcinoma the 5-year relative survival rates are 100% for stages I and II, 79.4% for stage III, and 47.1% for stage IV [31].

An estimate of a patient's risk profile may be used to decide between treatment approaches (lobectomy versus total thyroidectomy) in low-risk patients. Three of the best-known profiles are the AGES, AMES, and MACIS assessments, which have been mentioned previously.

## Summary

Recent advances in the postoperative care of patients with well-differentiated thyroid carcinoma allow more focused surveillance and the potential ability to identify patients requiring aggressive surgical intervention sooner. Surgical treatment options remain relatively unchanged.

## References

[1] Thyroid Carcinoma Task Force. AACE/AAES medical/surgical guidelines for clinical practice: management of thyroid carcinoma. American Association of Clinical Endocrinologists. American College of Endocrinology. Endocr Pract 2001;7:202–20.

[2] Ries LAG, Eisner MP, Kosary CL, et al, editors. SEER cancer statistics review, 1975–2001, National Cancer Institute. Bethesda, MD: National Cancer Institute. 2002. Available at: http://seer.cancer.gov/csr/1975_2001/, 2004. Accessed July 2003.

[3] Franceschi S, Boyle P, Maisonneuve P, et al. The epidemiology of thyroid carcinoma. Crit Rev Oncog 1993;4:25–52.

[4] Gillenwater AM, Weber RS. Thyroid carcinoma. Cancer Treat Res 1997;90:149–69.

[5] Braga-Basaria M, Ringel MD. Clinical review: beyond radioiodine: a review of potential new therapeutic approaches for thyroid carcinoma. J Clin Endocrinol Metab 2003;88:1947–60.

[6] National Comprehensive Cancer Network. Thyroid carcinoma. Clinical Practice Guidelines in Oncology. Version 1, 2003. Available at: www.nncn.org/. Accessed July 2003.

[7] Greenspan FS. Irradiation exposure and thyroid cancer. JAMA 1977;237:2089–91.

[8] DeGroot LJ, Reilly M, Pinnameneni K, Refetoff S. Retrospective and prospective study of radiation-induced thyroid disease. Am J Med 1983;74:852–62.

[9] Mazzaferri EL. Management of a solitary thyroid nodule. N Engl J Med 1993;328:553–9.

[10] Brander AE, Viikinkoski VP, Nickels JI, et al. Importance of thyroid abnormalities detected at US screening: a 5-year follow-up. Radiology 2000;215:801–6.

[11] Tomimori E, Pedrinola F, Cavaliere H, et al. Prevalence of incidental thyroid disease in a relatively low iodine intake area. Thyroid 1995;5:273–6.

[12] Brander A, Viikinkoski P, Voutilainen, et al. Clinical versus ultrasound examination of the thyroid gland in common clinical practice. J Clin Ultrasound 1992;20:37–42.

[13] Marqusee E, Benson CB, Frates MC, et al. Usefulness of ultrasonography in the management of nodular thyroid disease. Ann Intern Med 2000;133:696–700.

[14] McCall A, Jarosz H, Lawrence AM, et al. The incidence of thyroid carcinoma in solitary cold nodules and in multinodular goiters.. Surgery 1986;100:1128–32.

[15] Belfiore A, La Rosa GL, La Porta GA, et al. Cancer risk in patients with cold thyroid nodules: relevance of iodine intake, sex, age, and multinodularity. Am J Med 1992; 93:363–9.

[16] Papini E, Guglielmi R, Bianchini A, et al. Risk of malignancy in nonpalpable thyroid nodules: predictive value of ultrasound and color-Doppler features. J Clin Endocrinol Metab 2002;87:1941–6.

[17] Piromalli D, Martelli G, Del Prato I, et al. The role of fine-needle aspiration in diagnosis of thyroid nodules: analysis of 795 consecutive cases. J Surg Oncol 1992;50:247–50.

[18] Caraway NP, Sneige N, Samaan NA. Diagnostic pitfalls in thyroid fine-needle aspiration: a review of 394 cases. Diagn Cytopathol 1993;9:345–50.

[19] Baloch Z, LiVolsi VA, Jain P, et al. Role of repeat fine-needle aspiration biopsy (FNAB) in the management of thyroid nodules. Diagn Cytopathol 2003;29:203–6.

[20] Hamming JF, Goslings BM, van Steenis GJ, et al. The value of fine needle aspiration biopsy in patients with nodular thyroid disease divided into groups of suspicion of malignant neoplasms on clinical grounds. Arch Intern Med 1990;150:133–6.

[21] Chan BK, Desser TS, McDougall IR, et al. Common and uncommon sonographic features of papillary thyroid carcinoma. J Ultrasound Med 2003;22:1083–90.

[22] Takashima S, Fukuda H, Nomura N, et al. Thyroid nodules: re-evaluation with ultrasound. J Clin Ultrasound 1995;23:179–84.

[23] Hay ID, Klee GG. Thyroid cancer diagnosis and management. Clin Lab Med 1993;13: 725–34.

[24] Albareda M, Puig-Domingo M, Wengrowicz S, et al. Clinical forms of presentation and evolution of diffuse sclerosing variant of papillary carcinoma and insular variant of follicular carcinoma of the thyroid. Thyroid 1998;8:385–91.

[25] Chow SM, Chan JK, Law SC, et al. Diffuse sclerosing variant of papillary thyroid carcinoma—clinical features and outcome. Eur J Surg Oncol 2003;29:446–9.

[26] Segal K, Friedental R, Lubin E, et al. Papillary carcinoma of the thyroid. Otolaryngol Head Neck Surg 1995;113:356–63.

[27] Passler C, Prager G, Scheuba C, et al. Follicular variant of papillary thyroid carcinoma: a long-term follow-up. Arch Surg 2003;138:1362–6.

[28] Sanders LE, Cady B. Differentiated thyroid cancer: reexamination of risk groups and outcome of treatment. Arch Surg 1998;133:419–25.

[29] Lopez-Penabad L, Chiu AC, Hoff AO, et al. Prognostic factors in patients with Hurthle cell neoplasms of the thyroid. Cancer 2003;97:1186–94.

[30] Piersanti M, Ezzat S, Asa SL. Controversies in papillary microcarcinoma of the thyroid. Endocr Pathol 2003;14:183–91.

[31] Greene FL, Page DL, Fleming ID, et al, editors. American Joint Committee on Cancer cancer staging manual. 6th edition. New York: Springer Verlag; 2002.

[32] Hay ID, Grant CS, Taylor WF, et al. Ipsilateral lobectomy versus bilateral lobar resection in papillary thyroid carcinoma: a retrospective analysis of surgical outcome using a novel prognostic scoring system. Surgery 1987;102:1088–95.

[33] Shaha AR, Shah JP, Loree TR. Low-risk differentiated thyroid cancer: the need for selective treatment. Ann Surg Oncol 1997;4:328–33.

[34] Shah JP, Loree TR, Dharker D, et al. Lobectomy versus total thyroidectomy for differentiated carcinoma of the thyroid: a matched pair analysis. Am J Surg 1993;166: 331–5.

[35] Attie JN, Bock G, Moskowitz GW, et al. Postoperative radioactive evaluation of total thyroidectomy for thyroid carcinoma: reappraisal and therapeutic implications. Head Neck 1992;14:297–302.

[36] Gagel RF, Goepfert H, Callender DL. Changing concepts in the pathogenesis and management of thyroid carcinoma. CA 1996;46:261–83.

[37] Mazzaferri EL, Jhiang SM. Long-term impact of initial surgical and medical therapy on papillary and follicular thyroid cancer. Am J Med 1994;97:418–28.

[38] Samaan NA, Schultz PN, Hickey RC, et al. The results of various modalities of treatment of well-differentiated thyroid carcinoma: a retrospective review of 1599 patients. J Clin Endocrinol Metab 1992;75:714–20.

[39] Cady B, Rossi R. An expanded view of risk-group definition in differentiated thyroid carcinoma. Surgery 1988;104:947–53.

[40] Hay ID, Bergstralh EJ, Goellner JR, et al. Predicting outcome in papillary thyroid carcinoma: development of a reliable prognostic scoring system in a cohort of 1779 patients surgically treated at one institution during 1940 through 1989. Surgery 1993;114: 1050–8.

[41] Solomon BL, Wartofsky L, Burman KD. Current trends in the management of well-differentiated papillary thyroid carcinoma. J Clin Endocrin Metab 1996;81:333–9.

[42] Callcut RA, Selvaggi SM, Mack E, et al. The utility of frozen section evaluation for follicular thyroid lesions. Ann Surg Oncol 2004;11:94–8.

[43] Marcus B, Edwards B, Yoo S, et al. Recurrent laryngeal nerve monitoring in thyroid and parathyroid surgery: the University of Michigan experience. Laryngoscope 2003;113: 356–61.

[44] De Jong SA, Demeter JG, Lawrence AM, et al. Necessity and safety of completion thyroidectomy for differentiated thyroid carcinoma. Surgery 1992;112:734–9.

[45] Pasieka JL, Thompson NW, McLeod MK, et al. The incidence of bilateral well-differentiated thyroid cancer found at completion thyroidectomy. World J Surg 1992;16: 711–7.

[46] Kupferman ME, Mandel SJ, DiDonato L, et al. Safety of completion thyroidectomy following unilateral lobectomy for well-differentiated thyroid cancer. Laryngoscope 2002; 112:1209–12.

[47] McCaffrey TV, Bergstralh EJ, Hay ID. Locally invasive papillary thyroid carcinoma: 1940–1990. Head Neck 1994;16:165–72.

[48] McCaffrey TV, Lipton RJ. Thyroid carcinoma invading the upper aerodigestive system. Laryngoscope 1990;100:824–30.

[49] McHenry CR, Rosen IB, Walfish PG. Prospective management of nodal metastases in differentiated thyroid cancer. Am J Surg 1991;162:353–6.

[50] McCaffrey JC. Evaluation and treatment of aerodigestive tract invasion by well-differentiated thyroid carcinoma. Cancer Control 2000;7:246–52.

[51] Kowalski LP, Filho JG. Results of the treatment of locally invasive thyroid carcinoma. Head Neck 2002;24:340–4.

[52] Friedman M, Danielzadeh JA, Calderelli DD. Treatment of patients with carcinoma of the thyroid invading the airway. Arch Otolaryngol Head Neck Surg 1994;120:1377–81.

[53] Hammoud ZT, Mathisen DJ. Surgical management of thyroid carcinoma invading the trachea. Chest Surg Clin N Am 2003;13:359–67.

[54] Friedman M. Surgical management of thyroid carcinoma with laryngotracheal invasion. Otolaryngol Clin North Am 1990;23:495–507.

[55] Grillo HC, Suen HC, Mathisen DJ, et al. Resectional management of thyroid carcinoma invading the airway. Ann Thorac Surg 1992;54:3–10.

[56] Gillenwater AM, Goepfert H. Surgical management of laryngotracheal and esophageal involvement by locally advanced thyroid cancer. Semin Surg Oncol 1999;16:19–29.

[57] Falk SA, McCaffrey TV. Management of the recurrent laryngeal nerve in suspected and proven thyroid cancer. Otolaryngol Head Neck Surg 1995;113:42–8.

[58] Mizuno S, Funahashi H, Kondo A, et al. Regional lymph node metastasis in the early stage of thyroid cancer with special reference to the dissection method. Nagoya J Med Sci 1983;45: 71–7.

[59] Shaha AR. Management of the neck in thyroid cancer. Otolaryngol Clin North Am 1998;31: 823–31.

[60] Cady B, Rossi R, Silverman M, et al. Further evidence of the validity of risk group definition in differentiated thyroid carcinoma. Surgery 1985;98:1171–8.

[61] Sellers M, Beenken S, Blankenship A, et al. Prognostic significance of cervical lymph node metastases in differentiated thyroid cancer. Am J Surg 1992;164:578–81.

[62] Hughes CJ, Shaha AR, Shah JP, et al. Impact of lymph node metastasis in differentiated carcinoma of the thyroid: a matched-pair analysis. Head Neck 1996;18:127–32.

[63] Weber RS, Marvel J, Smith P, et al. Paratracheal lymph node dissection for carcinoma of the larynx, hypopharynx, and cervical esophagus. Otolaryngol Head Neck Surg 1993;108:11–7.

[64] Kupferman ME, Patterson DM, Mandel SJ, et al. Safety of modified radical neck dissection for differentiated thyroid carcinoma. Laryngoscope 2004;114:403–6.

[65] Robbins RJ, Tuttle RM, Sonenberg M, et al. Radioiodine ablation of thyroid remnants after preparation with recombinant human thyrotropin. Thyroid 2001;11:865–9.

[66] Sisson JC, Shulkin BL, Lawson S. Increasing efficacy and safety of treatments of patients with well-differentiated thyroid carcinoma by measuring body retentions of 131I. J Nucl Med 2003;44:898–903.

[67] Haugen BR, Pacini F, Reiners C, et al. A comparison of recombinant human thyrotropin and thyroid hormone withdrawal for the detection of thyroid remnant or cancer. J Clin Endocrinol Metab 1999;84:3877–85.

[68] Mazzaferri EL, Robbins RJ, Spencer CA, et al. A consensus report of the role of serum thyroglobulin as a monitoring method for low-risk patients with papillary thyroid carcinoma. J Clin Endocrinol Metab 2003;88:1433–41.

[69] Cohen EG, Tuttle RM, Kraus DH. Postoperative management of differentiated thyroid cancer. Otolaryngol Clin North Am 2003;36:129–57.

[70] Larson SM, Robbins R. Positron emission tomography in thyroid cancer management. Semin Roentgenol 2002;37:169–74.

[71] Pacini F, Agate L, Elisei R, et al. Outcome of differentiated thyroid cancer with detectable serum Tg and negative diagnostic (131) I whole body scan: comparison of patients treated with high (131) I activities versus untreated. J Clin Endocrinol Metab 2001;86:4092–7.

[72] Lowe VJ, Mullan BP, Hay ID, et al. 18F-FDG PET of patients with Hurthle cell carcinoma. J Nucl Med 2003;44:1402–6.

[73] Diehl M, Graichen S, Menzel C, et al. F-18 FDG PET in insular thyroid cancer. Clin Nucl Med 2003;28:728–31.

[74] Jadvar H, Fischman AJ. Evaluation of rare tumors with [F-18] fluorodeoxyglucose positron emission tomography. Clin Positron Imaging 1999;2:153–8.

[75] Brierley JD, Tsang RW. External-beam radiation therapy in the treatment of differentiated thyroid cancer. Semin Surg Oncol 1999;16:42–9.

[76] Pak H, Gourgiotis L, Chang W, et al. Role metastasectomy in the management of thyroid carcinoma: the NIH experience. J Surg Oncol 2003;82:10–8.

[77] Shoup M, Stojadinovic A, Nissan A, et al. Prognostic indicators of outcomes in patients with distant metastases from differentiated thyroid carcinoma. J Am Coll Surg 2003;197:191–7.

Otolaryngol Clin N Am
38 (2005) 179–184

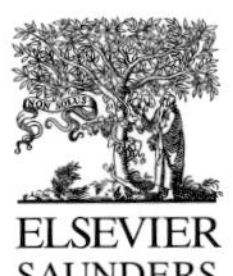

ELSEVIER
SAUNDERS

OTOLARYNGOLOGIC
CLINICS
OF NORTH AMERICA

# Index

*Note:* Page numbers of article titles are in **boldface** type.

# *Changing Your Address?*

Make sure your subscription changes too! When you notify us of your new
address, you can help make our job easier by including an exact copy of your
Clinics label number with your old address (see illustration below.) This
number identifies you to our computer system and will speed the processing of
your address change. Please be sure this label number accompanies your old
address and your corrected address—you can send an old Clinics label with
your number on it or just copy it exactly and send it to the address listed below.

We appreciate your help in our attempt to give you continuous coverage.
Thank you.

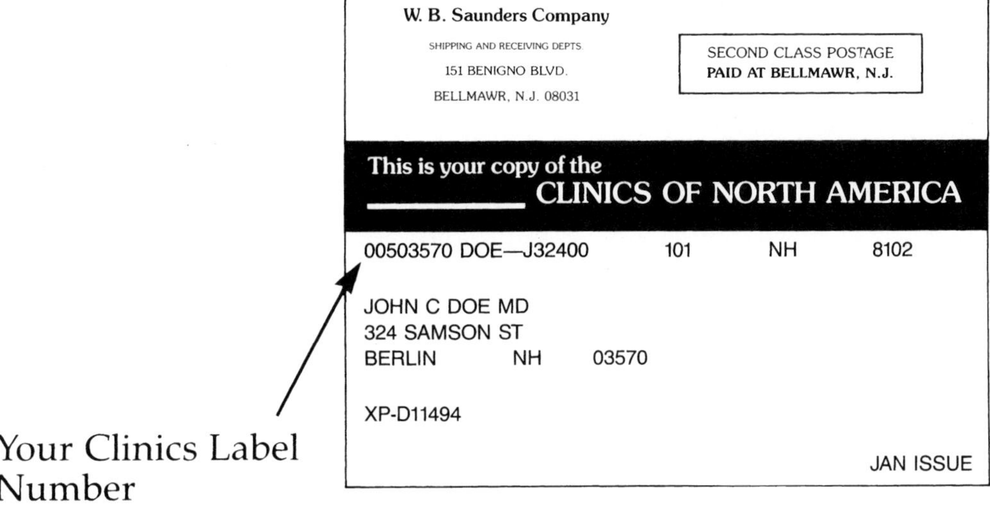



Your Clinics Label
Number
Copy it exactly or send your label
along with your address to:
**W.B. Saunders Company, Customer Service**
Orlando, FL 32887-4800
Call Toll Free 1-800-654-2452

Please allow four to six weeks for delivery of new subscriptions and for
processing address changes.